Management of Sepsis: The PIRO Approach

Jordi Rello • Emili Díaz • Alejandro Rodríguez (Eds.)

Management of Sepsis: The PIRO Approach

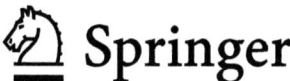

Editors
Jordi Rello, MD, PhD
Intensive Care Unit
Joan XXIII University Hospital
Carrer Mallafré Guasch, 4
43007 Tarragona
Spain
jrello.hj23.ics@gencat.cat

Emili Díaz, MD, PhD
Intensive Care Unit
Joan XXIII University Hospital
Carrer Mallafré Guasch, 4
43007 Tarragona
Spain
Emilio.diaz.santos@gmail.com

Alejandro Rodríguez, MD, PhD
Intensive Care Unit
Joan XXIII University Hospital
Carrer Mallafré Guasch, 4
43007 Tarragona
Spain
arodri.hj23.ics@gencat.cat

ISBN: 978-3-642-10148-9   e-ISBN: 978-3-642-00479-7
DOI: 10.1007/978-3-642-00479-7
Springer Dordrecht Heidelberg London New York

© Springer-Verlag Berlin Heidelberg 2010
This work is subject to copyright. All rights are reserved, whether the whole or part of the material is concerned, specifically the rights of translation, reprinting, reuse of illustrations, recitation, broadcasting, reproduction on microfilm or in any other way, and storage in data banks. Duplication of this publication or parts thereof is permitted only under the provisions of the German Copyright Law of September 9, 1965, in its current version, and permission for use must always be obtained from Springer. Violations are liable to prosecution under the German Copyright Law.
The use of general descriptive names, registered names, trademarks, etc. in this publication does not imply, even in the absence of a specific statement, that such names are exempt from the relevant protective laws and regulations and therefore free for general use.
Product liability: The publishers cannot guarantee the accuracy of any information about dosage and application contained in this book. In every individual case the user must check such information by consulting the relevant literature.

Cover design: eStudioCalamar, Spain

Printed on acid-free paper

Springer is part of Springer Science+Business Media (www.springer.com)

Contents

1. **PIRO: The Key to Success?** 1
   Jean-Louis Vincent

2. **Risk Stratification in Severe Sepsis: Organ Failure Scores or PIRO?** 11
   Rui P. Moreno, Ana Cristina Diogo, and Susana Afonso

3. **Community-Acquired Pneumonia Management Based on the PIRO System. A New Therapeutic Paradigm** 23
   Ignacio Martin-Loeches and Jordi Rello

4. **Ventilator-Associated Pneumonia PIRO Score** 39
   Emili Díaz and Thiago Lisboa

5. **A PIRO-Based Approach for Severity Assessment in Community-Acquired Pneumonia** 51
   Thiago Lisboa, Alejandro Rodríguez, and Jordi Rello

6. **Real-Time PCR in Microbiology: From Diagnosis to Characterization** 65
   Malte Book, Lutz Eric Lehmann, Xiang Hong Zhang, and Frank Stueber

7. **Influence of Serotype in Pneumococcal Disease: A New Challenge for Vaccination** 87
   Manel Luján, Yolanda Belmonte, and Dionisia Fontanals

8. **Acute Kidney Injury and Extracorporeal Blood Purification in Sepsis** 97
   Javier Maynar Moliner, José Ángel Sánchez-Izquierdo Riera, Manuel Herrera Gutiérrez, Amaia Quintano Rodero, and Alberto Manzano Ramirez

9. **Immunoglobulin, Sepsis, and Pneumonia** 117
   Jordi Almirall, Ester Vendrell, and Javier de Gracia

| 10 | Coagulation Disorders in Sepsis | 131 |

Marcel Schouten and Tom van der Poll

| 11 | Antibiotics in Severe Sepsis: Which Combinations Work? | 147 |

Tobias Welte

Index 159

Contributors

Susana Afonso
Unidade de Cuidados Intensivos
Polivalente
Hospital de St. António dos Capuchos
Centro Hospitalar de Lisboa Central E.P.E.
1150-069 Lisbon
Portugal

Jordi Almirall
Critical Care Unit
University Hospital de Mataró
University of Barcelona
CIBER Enfermedades Respiratorias
C/ Villaroel 170
08036 Barcelona
Spain
jalmirall@csdm.cat

Yolanda Belmonte
Department of Pneumology
Hospital de Sabadell
Parc Taulí, s/n.
08208 Sabadell
Spain

Malte Book
University Department
of Anaesthesiology
and Pain Therapy
Inselspital
3010 Bern
Switzerland
Malte.Book@dkf.unibe.ch

Emili Díaz
Critical Care Department
Joan XXIII University Hospital
University Rovira & Virgili
Institut Pere Virgili
CIBER Enfermedades Respiratorias
Carrer Doctor Mallafré Guasch, 4
43007 Tarragona
Spain
Emilio.diaz.santos@gmail.com

Ana Cristina Diogo
Unidade de Cuidados Intensivos Polivalente
Hospital de St. António dos Capuchos
Centro Hospitalar de Lisboa Central E.P.E.
1150-069 Lisbon
Portugal

Dionisia Fontanals
Department of Pneumology
Hospital de Sabadell
Parc Taulí, s/n.
08208 Sabadell
Spain

Javier de Gracia
Respiratory Intensive Care Unit
Pulmonary Department
University Hospital Vall d'Hebron
CIBER Enfermedades Respiratorias
C/Villaroel 170
08036 Barcelona
Spain

Manuel Herrera Gutiérrez
Department of Intensive Care Medicine
Carlos Haya Hospital
Avda. Carlos Haya, s/n
29010 Malaga
Spain

Lutz Eric Lehmann
Department of Anaesthesiology and
Intensive Care Medicine
University of Bonn
Sigmund-Freud-Str. 25
53105 Bonn
Germany
Lutz.Lehmann@ukb.uni-bonn.de

Thiago Lisboa
Critical Care Department
Joan XXIII University Hospital
University Rovira & Virgili
Institut Pere Virgili
CIBER Enfermedades Respiratorias
Carrer Doctor Mallafré Guasch, 4
43007 Tarragona
Spain
tlisboa@hotmail.com

Manel Luján
Department of Pneumology
Hospital de Sabadell
Parc Taulí, s/n.
08208 Sabadell
Spain
mlujan@tauli.cat

Ignacio Martin-Loeches
Critical Care Department
Joan XXIII University Hospital
University Rovira & Virgili
Institut Pere Virgili
CIBER Enfermedades Respiratorias
Carrer Doctor Mallafré Guasch, 4
43007 Tarragona
Spain

Alberto Manzano Ramirez
Department of Intensive Care Medicine
Santiago Apóstol Hospital
C/Olaguibel n° 29
01104 Vitoria
Spain

Rui P. Moreno
Unidade de Cuidados Intensivos
Polivalente
Hospital de St. António dos Capuchos
Centro Hospitalar de Lisboa Central E.P.E.
1150-069 Lisbon
Portugal
r.moreno@mail.telepac.pt

Amaia Quintano Rodero
Department of Intensive Care Medicine
Santiago Apóstol Hospital
C/Olaguibel n° 29
01104 Vitoria
Spain

Jordi Rello
Critical Care Department
Joan XXIII University Hospital
University Rovira i Virgili
Institut Pere Virgili
CIBER Enfermedades Respiratorias
Carrer Dr. Mallafré Guasch, 4
43007 Tarragona
Spain
jrello.hj23.ics@gencat.cat

Alejandro Rodríguez
Critical Care Department
Joan XXIII University Hospital
University Rovira i Virgili
Institut Pere Virgili
CIBER Enfermedades Respiratorias
Carrer Dr. Mallafré Guasch, 4
43007 Tarragona
Spain
arodri.hj23.ics@gencat.cat

José Ángel Sánchez-Izquierdo Riera
Department of Intensive Care Medicine
Doce de Octubre Hospital
C/Riaza 3, 2° D
28023 Madrid
Spain

Marcel Schouten
Center for Infection and Immunity
Amsterdam (CINIMA)
Center for Experimental and Molecular
Medicine (CEMM)
Academic Medical Center
University of Amsterdam
Meibergdreef 9, room G2-130
1105 AZ Amsterdam
The Netherlands

Javier Maynar Moliner
Department of Intensive Care Medicine
Santiago Apóstol Hospital
C/Olaguibel n° 29
01104 Vitoria
Spain
Franciscojavier.maynarmoliner@
osakidetza.net

Frank Stueber
University Department of Anaesthesiology
and Pain Therapy
Inselspital
3010 Bern
Switzerland
Frank.Stueber@insel.ch

Tom van der Poll
Center for Infection and Immunity
Amsterdam (CINIMA)
Center for Experimental and Molecular
Medicine (CEMM)
Academic Medical Center
University of Amsterdam
Meibergdreef 9, room G2-130
1105 AZ Amsterdam
The Netherlands
t.vanderpoll@amc.uva.nl

Ester Vendrell
Hospital Comarcal de Blanes
Accés Cala Sant Francesc 5
17300 Blanes (Girona)
Spain

Jean-Louis Vincent
Department of Intensive Care
Erasme Hospital
Université Libre de Bruxelles
Route de Lennik 808
1070 Brussels
Belgium
jlvincent@ulb.ac.be

Tobias Welte
Department of Respiratory Medicine
Medizinische Hochschule Hannover
Carl-Neuberg-Str. 1
30625 Hannover
Germany
Welte.tobias@mh-hannover.de

Xiang Hong Zhang
Department of Anaesthesiology and
Intensive Care Medicine
University of Bonn
Sigmund-Freud-Str. 25
53105 Bonn
Germany
zxh_820116@hotmail.com

PIRO: The Key to Success?

Jean-Louis Vincent

1
Background

Over the years, there has been considerable confusion regarding the definition of sepsis, with terms such as "infection" and "sepsis" often being used interchangeably. While obviously related, these elements are not exact synonyms; sepsis is the host response to an infection by an invading microorganism, be it virus, bacteria, or fungus. In 1992, as the links between inflammation and sepsis were becoming increasingly clear, a consensus conference on sepsis definitions introduced the term SIRS (systemic inflammatory response syndrome) in an attempt to clarify and simplify the definitions of sepsis [1]. A patient was classified as having SIRS if he/she had at least two of four parameters (temperature >38 or <36°C; heart rate >90 beats/min; respiratory rate >20 breaths per minute or PCO_2 < 32 mmHg; white blood cell count >12 or <4 × 10^9/l). Sepsis was defined as SIRS plus infection. However, it soon became apparent that nearly all intensive care unit (ICU) patients meet the SIRS criteria at some point during their ICU stay [2, 3], making this approach too sensitive to be useful in diagnosing sepsis [4].

Almost 10 years later, a second consensus conference on sepsis definitions was convened, sponsored by the Society of Critical Care Medicine (SCCM), the European Society of Intensive Care Medicine (ESICM), the American College of Chest Physicians (ACCP), the American Thoracic Society (ATS), and the Surgical Infection Societies (SIS) [5]. The participants at this meeting agreed that the SIRS concept was not helpful and should no longer be used per se, but that the SIRS criteria be incorporated into a longer list of signs of sepsis that could be employed to support a diagnosis of sepsis. This list includes biologic signs of inflammation (e.g., increased serum concentrations of C-reactive protein [CRP] or procalcitonin), hemodynamic parameters (e.g., increased cardiac output, low systemic vascular resistance [SVR], low oxygen extraction ratio), signs of altered tissue perfusion (e.g., altered skin perfusion, reduced urine output), and signs of organ dysfunction (e.g., increased urea and creatinine, low platelet count or other coagulation abnormalities,

---

J.-L. Vincent (✉)
Department of Intensive Care, Erasme Hospital, Université Libre de Bruxelles,
Route de Lennik 808, 1070 Brussels, Belgium
e-mail: jlvincen@ulb.ac.be

hyperbilirubinemia). The participants also suggested that as the definitions did not allow for precise characterization and staging of patients with sepsis, a clinically useful staging system that could stratify patients by both their baseline risk of an adverse outcome and their potential to respond to therapy was needed. Building on a system that had emerged at the Fifth Toronto Sepsis Roundtable held in Toronto, Canada, in 2000 [6], the sepsis definitions conference participants, therefore, proposed the PIRO system [5], which can classify patients on the basis of their *p*redisposing conditions, the nature and extent of the *i*nfection, the nature and magnitude of the host *r*esponse, and the degree of concomitant *o*rgan dysfunction.

2
Similarities Between Sepsis and Cancer

Disease stratifications systems are widely used in clinical medicine, but perhaps the most familiar and frequently employed is the TNM system, which was developed by Pierre Denoix in the 1940s [7], and is universally recognized as a standard for classifying patients with cancer. The TNM system classifies malignant tumors based on descriptors of the extent of the primary tumor (T), on the presence, absence, and extent of metastases to regional lymph nodes (N), and on the presence or absence of distant metastases (M) (Table 1). Each patient with a tumor will, therefore, receive a specific classification, e.g., T1, N0, M0, for that tumor. TNM classifications are then grouped into stages, usually from I to IV, which provide valuable prognostic information. Importantly, staging systems in cancer stratify patients not only according to prognosis, but also according to the probability that they will respond to a particular therapy.

Sepsis is in many ways very similar to cancer. Both disease processes are common, with high mortality rates. Both are the result of a complex pathophysiological process involving cellular dysregulation. Both can develop in (almost) any organ, and both frequently require surgical and medical therapies. Treatments for both are expensive and often involve several pharmacological agents. Finally, when treatment is successful, it is associated with slow step-by-step improvement.

Table 1 Basic TNM classification of cancers

Primary tumor (T)	
Tx	Primary tumor not evaluated
T0	No primary tumor
T1, 2, 3, 4	Size and/or extent of the primary tumor
Regional lymph nodes (N)	
Nx	Regional lymph nodes not evaluated
N0	No regional lymph node involvement
N1, 2, 3	Number and extent of regional lymph node involvement
Distant metastases (M)	
Mx	Distant metastases not evaluated
M0	No distant metastases
M1	Distant metastases

These similarities between sepsis and cancer led to the suggestion that a disease stratification system, similar to the TNM system for cancer, could be developed for sepsis [5]. The PIRO system for the grading of sepsis uses clinical and laboratory parameters to aid diagnosis and patient classification, with each element being divided according to the degree of involvement (e.g., infection can be classified as localized, extended, or generalized; immune response can be classified as limited, extensive, or excessive; organ dysfunction can be classified as mild, moderate, severe). As with the TNM system, it has been proposed that points could be allocated such that a patient with sepsis could, for example, be staged as $P_1I_2R_1O_0$ [6], depending on the features present for each of the four PIRO components.

3
PIRO Components

All aspects of the four components of the PIRO system impact on outcome and can influence therapeutic choices. As the TNM system is divided into clinical (cTcNcM) and pathological (pTpNpM) classifications, so each component of PIRO can be considered to have potentially relevant clinical and laboratory variables (Table 2).

3.1
Predisposition

Predisposition can include multiple factors such as age, sex, presence of certain premorbid diseases, prolonged immunosuppressant or antimicrobial medication, even cultural and religious beliefs [8]. All these factors individually and collectively can impact on outcome,

Table 2 Some suggested variables for the four components of the PIRO grading system

	Clinical	Laboratory
P: Predisposing factors	Age, coexisting diseases (alcoholism, diabetes, cirrhosis etc.), sex, steroid or immunosuppressive therapy	Genetic factors
I: Infection	Site (pneumonia, peritonitis, catheter), hospital acquired versus community-acquired	Bacteriology (infecting organism, virulence, sensitivity)
R: Response	Temperature, heart rate, blood pressure, cardiac output, etc	White blood cell count, prothrombin time, APTT, arterial blood gases, lactate levels, C-reactive protein, procalcitonin, other biomarkers
O: Organ dysfunction	Blood pressure, urine output, Glasgow Coma Scale	PaO_2/FiO_2, serum creatinine, serum bilirubin, platelet count

modifying both the disease process and the approach to therapy. Recent advances in genetic techniques have enabled several factors associated with an increased risk of infection and of mortality from sepsis to be identified. Single nucleotide polymorphisms, microsatellites, insertion and deletion polymorphisms are all forms of genetic variation that can characterize an individual's risk for sepsis, organ dysfunction, or death [9]. Most genetic traits associated with severe infection are associated with defects in innate immune responses. For example, a polymorphism of the tumor necrosis factor (TNF)-α gene, the TNF-2 allele, is associated with increased serum levels of TNF and a greater risk of mortality from septic shock [10]. A polymorphism within intron 2 of the interleukin-1 receptor antagonist (IL-1ra) gene (IL-1RN*2) has been associated with reduced IL-1ra production and increased mortality rates [11]. Recently, polymorphisms in the Toll-like receptor 1 gene were reported to be associated with increased susceptibility to organ dysfunction, death, and Gram-positive infection in sepsis [12].

Sex differences are another area of interest with several studies reporting that women are less likely to develop sepsis than men [13, 14]. However, women who do develop sepsis, particularly older women, may have worse outcomes than men [15, 16]. Studies have also suggested racial differences in susceptibility to and outcomes from sepsis [17], and older patients are known to be at an increased risk of developing sepsis and succumbing to it [18]. Certain chronic diseases, such as cirrhosis, diabetes, and chronic obstructive pulmonary disease (COPD), as well as chronic use of immunosuppressant medication may also predispose to sepsis and a worse outcome. Moreover, each factor may have a different impact on the other three PIRO components [5]. For example, chronic immunosuppression may increase a person's risk of infection, but may decrease the magnitude of that person's inflammatory response. Undoubtedly these are complex relationships with multiple confounding factors and further research is needed to clearly define which factors should be taken into account when considering the impact of predisposition on prognosis, to determine which carry most weight, and to identify how knowledge of increased risks can be translated into improved clinical outcomes. Advances in genetics technology now enable investigators to create glass slides (chips) with minute quantities of short, gene-specific nucleotides. These gene-specific probe nucleotides, ideally one for each gene in the genome, are arrayed onto the chip surface to produce a DNA microarray. These can be used to generate an expression profile, the transcriptome, for the cell or tissue of interest. Genomics, and the broader field of proteomics, is likely to be increasingly used in routine patient management in hospitals of the future and will facilitate the task of assessing predisposition.

3.2
Infection

Four key aspects related to the underlying infection can influence management and prognosis in patients with sepsis: source, degree, hospital-acquired versus community-acquired, and microorganism [19]. In terms of source, for example, infections of the urinary tract are usually less severe than intra-abdominal or pulmonary infections. In the Protein C Worldwide Evaluation in Severe Sepsis (PROWESS) trial [20], patients with urinary tract infections as a source of severe sepsis had a 28-day all-cause mortality of 21% compared with patients with a pulmonary source of sepsis who had a mortality rate of 34% ($p < .01$). The size of the inoculum, virulence, and sensitivity of the infecting organisms are also important in determining outcomes. In the Sepsis Occurrence in Acutely Ill Patients (SOAP) study, infection with *Pseudomonas spp.* was independently associated with increased ICU mortality (OR: 1.62 [95% CI 1.09–2.42], $p = 0.017$) [16]. In a multicenter study from China, Gram-positive bacterial infection and invasive fungal infections were risk factors for hospital mortality [21]. However, classifying the relative importance of infections on outcome can be difficult. Cohen et al. [22] recently generated specific risk codes for the six most common infections: bacteremia, meningitis, pneumonia, skin and soft tissue infections, peritonitis, and urinary tract infections. For each infection site and organism, a two-digit code was generated according to the mortality rate associated with that infection (from 1: ≤5% to 4: >30%), and the level of evidence available to support the mortality risk (level A representing evidence from more than five studies with greater than 100 patients, through to level E where there was insufficient evidence from case reports). This Grading System for Site and Severity of Infection (GSSSI) needs to be validated, but could be a useful means of characterizing the risks associated with infections caused by various organisms in different sites.

The timing of the onset of infection may also influence outcomes. One study showed that patients who developed septic shock within 24 h of ICU admission were more severely ill, but had better outcomes, than patients who became hypotensive later during their ICU stay [23].

3.3
Immune Response

Sepsis is defined as the host response to infection, yet that host response has proved difficult to characterize [24]. Various approaches have been proposed, including the presence of characteristic signs and symptoms or the degree of elevation of biological markers, such as procalcitonin or C-reactive protein, but as yet, none of the suggested markers is specific for sepsis. Importantly, the initial theory that sepsis was simply an uncontrolled inflammatory response and could be treated by blocking or removing any or several of the proinflammatory cytokines has been replaced by the realization that the inflammatory response is a normal and necessary response to infection, and interrupting that response at any point may do more harm than good. Indeed, the early hyperinflammatory phase of sepsis is soon replaced by a hypoinflammatory state. The host response to infection thus varies between patients and with time in the same patient [25]. This differentiation is important for therapeutic decisions, as antiinflammatory therapies may be harmful if given to a patient who is already in the hypoinflammatory phase; such a patient may benefit rather from a proinflammatory therapy to boost their immune system. As with genomics, technological advances now enable multiple markers to be assessed simultaneously from small blood samples. This approach could provide clinicians with an immune profile for individual patients. Again, considerable research is needed to indentify which markers should be included on such microarrays. Furthermore, the optimal set of biologic markers for any patient may depend on the therapy being proposed [5]. For example, an indicator of dysregulation of the coagulation system might be more valuable when deciding whether or not to give drotrecogin alfa (activated), whereas a marker of adrenal dysfunction might be more useful for determining whether to give hydrocortisone.

3.4
Organ Dysfunction

Organ dysfunction in severe sepsis is not a simple "present" or "absent" variable, but presents a continuous spectrum of varying severity in different organs over time [26]. The degree of organ involvement can be assessed with various scoring systems, such as the Sequential Organ Failure Assessment (SOFA) [27]. This system uses parameters that are routinely available in all ICUs to assess the degree of dysfunction for six organ systems: respiratory, cardiovascular, renal, coagulation, neurologic, and hepatic, with a scale of 0 (no dysfunction) to 4 for each organ. Importantly, organ dysfunction can be recorded for each organ separately or a composite score can be calculated. Thus with repeated scores, a dynamic picture of the effects of sepsis on individual or global organ dysfunction can be developed. Sequential assessment of the SOFA score during the first few days of ICU admission has been shown to be a good indicator of prognosis, with an increase in SOFA score during the first 48 h in the ICU predicting a mortality rate of at least 50% [28]. Levy et al. reported that early improvement in cardiovascular, renal, or respiratory function from baseline to day 1 was significantly related to survival [29]. Continued improvement in cardiovascular function before the start of day 2 and start of day 3 was associated with further improvement in survival for patients who improved compared with those who worsened.

In the future, organ dysfunction scores may be replaced by or combined with more direct assessment of cellular stress and injury, for example, measures of mitochondrial dysfunction, apoptosis, or cytopathic hypoxia.

4
PIRO in Practice

The PIRO concept at its simplest provides a means of putting some order to the various aspects of sepsis. Further work is needed to determine exactly which factors should be included in each of the four components and whether or how they should be measured and weighted to achieve a quantitative measure by which heterogeneous groups of septic patients could be characterized and categorized. Once validated, it is possible that patients could receive a PIRO grade or stage, e.g., $P_3I_2R_1O_2$, which would help direct treatment and indicate prognosis. In addition to characterizing individual patients, such grades would facilitate comparison of patient populations for clinical trial purposes and help focus clinical research.

Several groups have already attempted to apply the PIRO system clinically and the results of these studies will be discussed in more detail in later chapters. Moreno et al. used the SAPS III database to assess whether the PIRO system could be useful for predicting mortality in patients with sepsis [30]. For each of the four PIRO components, multivariate analysis was used to select variables significantly associated with hospital mortality, which were then weighted and allocated points. The authors felt it was not possible to separate host response from the resulting organ dysfunction, so they combined these two components. For predisposition, the final variables were age, location of patient prior to ICU admission, length of stay before ICU admission, certain comorbidities (cancer, cirrhosis, acquired immunodeficiency syndrome [AIDS]), and cardiac arrest as the reason for ICU admission; for infection, the variables were nosocomial infection, respiratory infection, and infections by *Candida* species or other fungi; for response/organ dysfunction, the variables were renal or coagulation dysfunction, and failure of the cardiovascular, renal, respiratory, coagulation, or central nervous systems. The authors suggested that, although further prospective validation is needed, the proposed SAPS III PIRO system could be used to stratify patients at or shortly after ICU admission to enable better selection of management according to the risk of death [30].

In a prospective, observational study, Lisboa et al. [31] applied the PIRO concept to patients with ventilator-associated pneumonia (VAP), again using multivariate logistic regression to identify variables independently associated with ICU mortality for inclusion in the PIRO model. In this study in VAP patients, the variables for predisposition were comorbidities (COPD, immunocompromise, heart failure, cirrhosis, chronic renal failure); for infection, the variable was bacteremia; for response, the variable was systolic blood pressure <90 mmHg; and for organ dysfunction, the variable was acute respiratory distress syndrome (ARDS). A four-point score was thus developed, with one point for each component. Mortality increased with increasing score: A score of 0 was associated with a mortality rate of 9.8%, increasing to 93.3% for patients with a score of 4. These authors suggested that the VAP-PIRO score could thus be a useful practical tool to predict disease severity in patients with VAP.

The two studies discussed briefly above are just two clinical examples of how the PIRO system could be adopted for use clinically.

5
Conclusion: Could PIRO Be the Key to Success?

Mortality remains high in patients with severe sepsis (around 40%) and septic shock (around 60%) and is closely associated with the degree of multiple organ failure. Results from studies of proposed new interventions in severe sepsis have largely been disappointing with few demonstrating any positive effect on outcomes. One of the possible reasons for the multiple "failed" trials is that the groups of patients studied have been too heterogeneous and that global results have masked any potential benefit in specific subgroups of patients [32]. Better targeting of proposed interventions by better characterization of septic patients with the PIRO system may lead to better outcomes. Improved classification of septic patients using the PIRO system may, thus, facilitate the development and evaluation of clinical trials of sepsis therapies and will also encourage further study into the pathophysiology and epidemiology of sepsis. Importantly, just as the TNM system is adjusted to specific cancers [33], so the PIRO system will need to be adapted to fit specific patient groups, local practice, purpose (e.g., clinical trial inclusion, prognostication, patient management), or proposed therapies. For example, if the planned intervention is an anticoagulant then evidence of coagulopathy is likely to be more relevant than presence of respiratory failure, while if considering hemodialysis, the presence and degree of renal failure are likely to be most pertinent [24].

However, despite general acceptance of the PIRO concept and belief that it may contribute to improving outcomes in patients with sepsis, many questions remain unanswered. For example, in patients with cancer, correct staging is critical because treatment is directly related to disease stage. Thus, incorrect staging can lead to improper treatment and to reduced patient outcomes. Whether the same would hold true for patients with sepsis is unknown. Clearly, considerable work remains to be done in testing and validating the PIRO system, but it represents an important step toward more successful management of the patient with severe sepsis.

References

1. ACCP-SCCM Consensus Conference (1992) Definitions of sepsis and multiple organ failure and guidelines for the use of innovative therapies in sepsis. Crit Care Med 20:864–874
2. Pittet D, Rangel-Frausto S, Li N, et al. (1995) Systemic inflammatory response syndrome, sepsis, severe sepsis and septic shock: incidence, morbidities and outcomes in surgical ICU patients. Intensive Care Med 21:302–309
3. Salvo I, de Cian W, Musicco M, et al. (1995) The Italian SEPSIS study: Preliminary results on the incidence and evolution of SIRS, sepsis, severe sepsis and septic shock. Intensive Care Med 21:S244–S249
4. Vincent JL (1997) Dear Sirs, I'm sorry to say that I don't like you. Crit Care Med 25: 372–374
5. Levy MM, Fink MP, Marshall JC, et al. (2003) 2001 SCCM/ESICM/ACCP/ATS/SIS International Sepsis Definitions Conference. Crit Care Med 31:1250–1256
6. Marshall JC, Vincent JL, Fink MP, et al. (2003) Measures, markers, and mediators: toward a staging system for clinical sepsis. A report of the Fifth Toronto Sepsis Roundtable, Toronto, Ontario, Canada, October 25–26, 2000. Crit Care Med 31:1560–1567
7. Denoix P (1946) Enquete permanent dans les centres anticancereaux. Bull Inst Natl Hyg 1:70–75
8. Angus DC, Burgner D, Wunderink R, et al. (2003) The PIRO concept: P is for predisposition. Crit Care 7:248–251
9. Cobb JP, O'Keefe GE (2004) Injury research in the genomic era. Lancet 363:2076–2083
10. Appoloni O, Dupont E, Andrien M, et al. (2001) Association of TNF2, a TNFα promoter polymorphism, with plasma TNFα levels and mortality in septic shock. Am J Med 110:486–488
11. Arnalich F, Lopez-Maderuelo D, Codoceo R, et al. (2002) Interleukin-1 receptor antagonist gene polymorphism and mortality in patients with severe sepsis. Clin Exp Immunol 127:331–336
12. Wurfel MM, Gordon AC, Holden TD, et al. (2008) Toll-like receptor 1 polymorphisms affect innate immune responses and outcomes in sepsis. Am J Respir Crit Care Med 178:710–720
13. Wichmann MW, Inthorn D, Andress HJ, Schildberg FW (2000) Incidence and mortality of severe sepsis in surgical intensive care patients: the influence of patient gender on disease process and outcome. Intensive Care Med 26:167–172

14. Martin GS, Mannino DM, Eaton S, Moss M (2003) The epidemiology of sepsis in the United States from 1979 through 2000. N Engl J Med 348:1546–1554
15. Romo H, Amaral AC, Vincent JL (2004) Effect of patient sex on intensive care unit survival. Arch Intern Med 164:61–65
16. Vincent JL, Sakr Y, Sprung CL, et al. (2006) Sepsis in European intensive care units: results of the SOAP study. Crit Care Med 34:344–353
17. Barnato AE, Alexander SL, Linde-Zwirble WT, Angus DC (2008) Racial variation in the incidence, care, and outcomes of severe sepsis: analysis of population, patient, and hospital characteristics. Am J Respir Crit Care Med 177:279–284
18. Martin GS, Mannino DM, Moss M (2006) The effect of age on the development and outcome of adult sepsis. Crit Care Med 34:15–21
19. Vincent JL, Opal S, Torres A, et al. (2003) The PIRO concept: I is for infection. Crit Care 7:252–255
20. Bernard GR, Vincent JL, Laterre PF, et al. (2001) Efficacy and safety of recombinant human activated protein C for severe sepsis. N Engl J Med 344:699–709
21. Cheng B, Xie G, Yao S, et al. (2007) Epidemiology of severe sepsis in critically ill surgical patients in ten university hospitals in China. Crit Care Med 35:2538–2546
22. Cohen J, Cristofaro P, Carlet J, Opal S (2004) New method of classifying infections in critically ill patients. Crit Care Med 32:1510–1526
23. Roman-Marchant O, Orellana-Jimenez CE, De Backer D, et al. (2004) Septic shock of early or late onset: does it matter? Chest 126:173–178
24. Gerlach H, Dhainaut JF, Harbarth S, et al. (2003) The PIRO Concept: R is for response. Crit Care 7:256–259
25. Volk HD, Reinke P, Krausch D, et al. (1996) Monocyte deactivation – rationale for a new therapeutic strategy in sepsis. Intensive Care Med 22:S474–S481
26. Vincent JL, Wendon J, Groeneveld J, et al. (2003) The PIRO concept: O is for organ dysfunction. Crit Care 7:260–264
27. Vincent JL, de Mendonça A, Cantraine F, et al. (1998) Use of the SOFA score to assess the incidence of organ dysfunction/failure in intensive care units: Results of a multicentric, prospective study. Crit Care Med 26:1793–1800
28. Lopes Ferreira F, Peres Bota D, Bross A, et al. (2001) Serial evaluation of the SOFA score to predict outcome. JAMA 286:1754–1758
29. Levy MM, Macias WL, Vincent JL, et al. (2005) Early changes in organ function predict eventual survival in severe sepsis. Crit Care Med 33:2194–2201
30. Moreno RP, Metnitz B, Adler L, et al. (2008) Sepsis mortality prediction based on predisposition, infection and response. Intensive Care Med 34:496–504
31. Lisboa T, Diaz E, Sa-Borges M, et al. (2008) The ventilator-associated pneumonia PIRO score: a tool for predicting ICU mortality and health-care resources use in ventilator-associated pneumonia. Chest 134:1208–1216
32. Vincent JL, Sun Q, Dubois MJ (2002) Clinical trials of immunomodulatory therapies in severe sepsis and septic shock. Clin Infect Dis 34:1084–1093
33. Sobin LH, Wittekind C (2002) TNM Classification of Malignant Tumours, 6th ed. Hoboken: Wiley

Risk Stratification in Severe Sepsis: Organ Failure Scores or PIRO?

Rui P. Moreno, Ana Cristina Diogo, and Susana Afonso

"It's more important to know what sort of person this disease has, than what sort of disease this person has"

William Osler, 1849–1919

1 Introduction

In the mid-1980s, a long series of clinical trials on patients with sepsis that yielded negative results started a very interesting discussion on the robustness of 28-day all-cause mortality as the sole or major end point for the evaluation of clinical trials in intensive care units (ICUs) [1]. The use of this measure, considered the gold standard in clinical trials on sepsis, undoubtedly represents a very relevant end point. It has, however, been contested [2], since hospital policy can and does change the location of deaths (e.g., discharging patients to die) and can be significantly underestimated in hospitals that discharge patients very early in the course of their disease. Moreover, the process of using two groups of patients, with one assigned to receive the new therapy and the other placebo, has been criticized. The absence of stratification according to patient demographic or biological characteristics before randomization can lead to unbalanced groups and confounding, and an impossibly high number of patients would be needed to demonstrate a significant difference between patient groups. In addition, interactions between certain patient characteristics at baseline and the effect of treatment can be obscured, as occurred in the MONARCS trial, in which the administration of afelimomab lowered the circulating levels of tumor necrosis factor (TNF) and interleukin (IL)-6, accelerated the resolution of organ dysfunction, and reduced 28-day all-cause mortality, but only in patients with elevated IL-6 levels at baseline [3].

For these reasons, some investigators have proposed certain recommendations that should constitute the basis of criteria for inclusion in clinical trials and that should not be restricted to the ones proposed by the American College of Chest Physicians (ACCP)/Society of Critical Care Medicine (SCCM) definitions of sepsis or sepsis syndrome. Moreover, they also proposed

R.P. Moreno (✉)
Unidade de Cuidados Intensivos Polivalente, Hospital de St. António dos Capuchos,
Centro Hospitalar de Lisboa Central E.P.E., 1150-069 Lisbon, Portugal
e-mail: r.moreno@mail.telepac.pt

the use of a scoring system for organ dysfunctions that has been validated and that can be incorporated into all sepsis studies. Furthermore, they recommend that generally the primary outcome measure should be mortality rate, but under appropriate circumstances major morbidities could be considered also as primary end points [4]. The publication in March 2001 of the Efficacy and Safety of Recombinant Human Activated Protein C for Severe Sepsis (PROWESS) trial presented apparently a decrease in 28-day all-cause mortality from 30.8% in the placebo group to 24.7% in the drotrecogin alfa-activated group [5]. However, it was soon evident that there were innumerous confounders and effect modifiers on the effect of the drug on patient outcome, of which the baseline severity of illness and site of infection were described as the most important [5, 6]. These potential confounding factors, and the later publication of studies with discrepant results in controlled [7] and uncontrolled settings [8, 9] raised such a serious debate [10] that the drug is now being assessed in a risk-stratified population [11].

In another more recent study, the CORTICUS study [12], comparing the use of hydrocortisone with placebo in patients with septic shock, baseline severity of illness and possibly other baseline and infection-related factors played such an important role in the interpretation of the results that they could be responsible for the negative result of the intervention on 28-day all-cause mortality, when compared with almost the same study design in a cohort of more severely ill patients [13]. This effect was even more striking because, although there was no change in 28-day all-cause mortality, there was clearly a reduction in the length of shock and the severity of multiple organ dysfunction/failure syndrome (MODS), driven by an improvement of cardiovascular dysfunction/failure [14].

Authors like Petros, more than 10 years ago, began to question the adequacy of all cause-mortality as an end point [15]. A meaningful end point can only be chosen when a direct relationship between an event and its consequences is known. In the case of sepsis (and multiple organ failure) our knowledge is very limited, and concerning most phenomena no such direct relationship can be established. Moreover, it implies the need for large samples, with problems in reliability of data collection, heterogeneity of enrolled patients, and costs. Patients in intensive care, even with strict inclusion criteria for sepsis or septic shock, do not constitute a homogeneous sample. Patients have different syndromes and diagnoses, time-courses, ages, chronic illnesses (chronic health, comorbidities), different sites of infection and invading microorganisms, and different degrees of physiologic dysfunction resulting in a large diversity of mortality risks [16, 17]. Several methods have been proposed to deal with this variation [17–19], but they usually involve complex, extensive (and expensive) data collection and sophisticated analysis.

Two approaches have been designed to cope with this complex problem of patient selection and stratification, which have led to the development of the MODS scores and the so-called PIRO approach (predisposition, insult, response, and organ dysfunction).

2
Organ Dysfunction/Failure Scores

Awareness of the importance of MODS as an important confounder and/or effect modifier in the evaluation of patients with sepsis led the Working Group on Sepsis-Related Problems of the European Society of Intensive Care Medicine (ESICM), under the leadership of Professor

Jean-Louis Vincent, to organize a consensus meeting in Paris (December 1994) to create the so-called Sepsis-related Organ Failure Assessment (SOFA) score [20]. The rationale behind this decision was the need to find an objective and simple way to describe individual organ dysfunction/failure in a continuous form, from mild dysfunction to severe failure, which could be used over time to measure the evolution of individual (or aggregated) organ dysfunction in clinical trials on sepsis or by the clinician at the bedside. A retrospective evaluation of the application of this score in the first 24 h after ICU admission on 1,643 patients with early sepsis in an international database [20] demonstrated a good correlation with mortality and an acceptable distribution of the patients among the different groups. To confirm these retrospective findings, a prospective, multinational study was initiated that demonstrated that the system could in fact be applied in other typologies of patients and for this reason the name of the score was changed to Sequential Organ Failure Score.

Later, more complex measures were derived from this concept, such as the total maximum SOFA score and delta SOFA score (total maximum SOFA minus admission total SOFA, i.e., the magnitude of organ dysfunction appearing during the ICU stay), and they were shown to be even better as descriptors and/or predictors of outcome in patients with MODS (most of them septic) in ICUs all over the world [21].

Other similar systems exist, developed at more or less the same time, such as the MODS, created by Marshall and coworkers [22], and the Logistic Organ Dysfunction (LOD) system, developed by Le Gall and colleagues [23]. All of them were designed with similar principles in mind [20]:

(a) Organ failure is not a simple all-or-nothing phenomenon, it is a spectrum or continuum of organ dysfunction from very mild altered function to total organ failure.
(b) Organ failure is not a static process and the degree of dysfunction varies with time during the course of the disease.
(c) The variables chosen to evaluate each organ need to be objective, simple, and available but also reliable, routinely measured in every institution, specific to the organ in question, and independent of other disease-specific variables, so that the score can be easily calculated for any patient in any ICU.

Although there is no general agreement on the optimal way to assess organ dysfunction/failure, all the widely used systems include six key organ systems (cardiovascular, respiratory, hematological, central nervous, renal, and hepatic), evaluated through a combination of physiologic (e.g., PaO_2) and therapeutic (e.g., use of vasopressor agents) variables. The major difference among them is the method chosen for the evaluation of cardiovascular dysfunction: SOFA uses blood pressure and the level of adrenergic support, MODS uses a composed variable (pressure-adjusted heart rate or PAR = heart rate × central venous pressure/mean arterial pressure), and the LOD score uses the heart rate and systolic blood pressure. A comparison of these systems, published only as an abstract, seem to indicate a greater discriminative capability of the MODS and SOFA score over the LOD score [24]. However, the small size of the sample requires further validation.

Mixed models, integrating organ failure assessment scores and general severity scores, have been published [25, 26] but they have not gained widespread acceptance.

3
From Multiple Organ Dysfunction/Failure Scores to the PIRO Concept

In 2001, several European and American critical care societies organized a second consensus conference to address the weaknesses of systemic inflammatory response syndrome (SIRS) and sepsis definitions, discussed intensively over the last decade [27], with the aim of improving the early identification and stratification of patients with sepsis [28]. The result of this conference was the adoption of systemic inflammatory response syndrome as a broader definition of inflammation. Furthermore, minor changes were added to the definition of severe sepsis and septic shock. A new system for risk stratification, which emerged from the Fifth Toronto Sepsis Roundtable, held in Toronto, Canada in October 2000 [29], was also adopted: the IRO system (insult, response, and organ dysfunction), which later became the PIRO at the 2001 conference (with the addition of predisposition) [30–33]. Although interesting and promising, to date this approach has remained virtually conceptual, with the first attempt to develop such a system being just published as an abstract [34].

In the last few years, our group has empirically tested – using a large multicenter, multinational database, the Simplified Acute Physiology Score (SAPS) 3 database [35] – whether a modified definition of PIRO (using the concept of predisposition, infection, and response/organ dysfunction/failure) could be useful for predicting mortality in patients with severe infection, sepsis, and septic shock at ICU admission.

In this cohort (comprising 16,784 patients from 303 ICUs), 3,505 patients already presented an infection at ICU admission, from which 2,628 patients had a length of stay in the ICU equal to or greater than 48 h.

To test the PIRO concept, three logical boxes were defined:

(a) *Predisposition*: The variables of the SAPS 3 "Admission Score Boxes 1 and 2", which are not related to infection, were used. These include age, comorbidities, use of vasoactive drugs before ICU admission, intrahospital location before ICU admission, length of stay in the hospital before ICU admission, reason(s) for ICU admission, planned/unplanned ICU admission, surgical status at ICU admission and, if applicable, the anatomic site of surgery.
(b) *Infection*: For this box, all variables related to infection at ICU admission were used. These include acquisition of the infection, extension and site of infection, the presence of bacteremia, and the microbial agents identified.
(c) *Response/Organ dysfunction/Organ failure*: To identify the response and the consequences of the infection, we used the development of organ dysfunction and failure, measured through the highest SOFA score values for each organ system between admission and 48 h after ICU admission.

These variables were selected according to their association with hospital mortality as described elsewhere and a multilevel model (logistic regression with random effects) was applied, using patient characteristics as fixed effects and ICUs as a random effect, to estimate the impact of each of the predictive variables in the outcome variable [36].

In the multivariate analysis, the variables that turned out to be significant were:

(a) *Predisposition (Box 1)*: age; location from which the patient was admitted to the ICU; comorbidities; length of stay before ICU admission (days); and some reasons for ICU admission
(b) *Infection (Box 2)*: acquisition of infection; extension of infection; site of infection; and infective agent
(c) *Response/Organ dysfunction/Organ failure (Box 3)*: dysfunction of the renal and coagulation systems; failure of the cardiovascular, respiratory, renal, coagulation and central nervous systems

Based on the contribution of these variables to outcome, a score sheet was developed (Table 1) and an equation relating the SAPS 3 PIRO score to the vital status at hospital discharge was created:

$$\text{logit} = -46.6757 + \ln(\text{SAPS 3-PIRO} + 76.7688) * 9.8797$$

with the probability of hospital mortality being given by the equation:

$$\text{Probability of death} = \frac{e^{\text{logit}}}{1 + e^{\text{logit}}}.$$

The prognostic performance of the developed model was tested by means of discrimination and calibration and was found to be excellent, both in the overall population and in specific subgroups of patients, as defined by the ACCP/SCCM classification of sepsis and septic shock [36].

It should be noted that in this system, the evaluation of the response and the resultant organ dysfunction/failure has been collapsed. This happens because, in our understanding, the host response to the insult and the resulting organ dysfunction cannot be distinguished from each other based on clinical variables, and there are no specific biomarkers available and ready for clinical use that can do this. Therefore, this resulted in the proposed three-level staging model consisting of predisposition, infection, and response/organ dysfunction/failure. We anticipate that as new biomarkers or panels of biomarkers become available in the future, we will be able to differentiate, in the clinical setting, between true biological response and the physiological and pathological consequences of that response, the dysfunction and/or failure of the different body systems.

4
One PIRO or Many PIROs?

In the last few years, Jordi Rello and the Intensive Care Group from Tarragona have also proposed two models based on the PIRO concept, one for ventilator-associated pneumonia (VAP-PIRO) [37] and the other for community-acquired pneumonia (CAP-PIRO) [38]. Both are discussed in Chap. 4 of this book by Emili Diaz and Thiago Lisboa this volume.

Table 1 Scoresheet for computation of SAPS 3-PIRO. Adapted from Moreno et al. [36], with permission

	0	4	5	6	7	8	9	10	11
Box 1: predisposition									
Age, years	<40	>=40 <60				>=60 <70			>=70 <75
Location from which the pat. was admitted to the ICU		Same hospital							
Co-Morbidities				Cancer[a]		Cirrhosis[b]	AIDS[c]		
Length of stay before ICU admission, days	<14		>=14 <28		>=28				
Reason(s) for ICU admission							Cardiac arrest[d]		
Box 2: infection	0	4	5		7	8	9	10	11
Acquisition		Nosocomial[e]							
Extension		Other than localized[f]							
Site			Respiratory[g]						
Agent								Candida, Fungi[h]	
Box 3: response/ organ function	0	4	5		7	8	9	10	11
Organ dysfunction (OD)[j]		Renal	Coagulation						
Organ failure (OF)[j,k]			Cardiovascular				CNS		
			Respiratory				Coagulation		
							Renal		

[a] *Cancer* refers to the presence of: metastatic cancer, haematological cancer, chemotherapy, immunosupression other, radiotherapy, steroid treatment. Data definitions are presented in Appendix C of the ESM: Co-Morbidities: AIDS [36]

[b] *Cirrhosis* refers to the data definitions in Appendix C of the ESM: Co-Morbidities: AIDS [36]

[c] *AIDS* refers to the data definitions in Appendix C of the ESM: Co-Morbidities: AIDS [36]

[d] *Cardiac Arrest* refers to the data definitions in Appendix C of the ESM: Reasons for ICU Admission: Cardiovascular – Cardiac Arrest [36]

[e] *Nosocomial* refers to the data definitions in Appendix C of the ESM: Acute Infection at ICU Adrission – Acquisition: Hospital-Acquired [36]

[f] *Other than localized* refers to the data definitions in Appendix C of the ESM: Acute Infection at ICU Adrission – Localized infection with regional involvement, disseminated [36]

[g] *Respiratory* refers to the data definition in Appendix C of the ESM: Acute Infection at ICU Admission - Site: Lower Respiratory Tract: Pneumonia, Lung Abscess, Other [36]

[h] *Candida, fungi* refer to the data definitions in Appendix C of the ESM: Acute Infection at ICU Admission – Agent and Bacteremia: if any of the following was present in any of the fields: *Candida albicans*; Candida spp, other; fungi, other; [36]

[i] If the maximum SOFA value of day 1 and day 2 is 1 or 2

[j] If the maximum SOFA value of day 1 and day 2 is 3 or 4

[k] With multiple items the points are additive

Both systems are very simple and share common characteristics:

(a) Developed in large cohorts of patients with community-acquired pneumonia requiring ICU admission and ventilator-associated pneumonia
(b) Computed at 24 h after ICU admission
(c) Use a simple scale comprising only a few variables (eight for CAP-PIRO and four for VAP-PIRO), derived by multivariate logistic regression with outcome at 28 days after ICU admission (CAP-PIRO) or vital status at ICU discharge (VAP-PIRO) used to select the variables
(d) Divide the patients into a few levels of risk (four for CAP-PIRO and three for VAP-PIRO) but do not provide a quantitative estimate of vital status at hospital discharge

These systems have the advantage over SAPS-PIRO of being easier to compute and more specific to the individual risk factors of the analyzed infections (CAP and VAP), but at the price of losing their applicability in large, more heterogeneous groups of patients with severe infection, sepsis, and septic shock. Moreover, they were derived from national, datasets and the extent of their utility outside the dataset demographics is unknown.

We hope that in the future a mixed approach can be used, creating a system that differentiates between general predisposition to severe infection and specific risk factors for specific infections, the characteristics of these infections, and the resulting organ dysfunction/failures impacting the outcome.

5
PIRO or MODS Scores?

The incidence of severe sepsis and septic shock in the ICU seems to be increasing in the last few years. This fact was consistently found in all recently published studies [39–42]. Although this trend can be partially explained by the growing awareness of physicians of the early recognition and treatment of sepsis as a result of initiatives such as the Surviving Sepsis Campaign [43], the increasing incidence seems to have been present even before these initiatives, and thus other reasons, such as the changing demographics of the population (increasing age, comorbidities) and the changing characteristics of the microorganisms (prevalence, resistance), probably play a major role in this phenomenon.

Although mortality in sepsis seems to be associated mainly with the presence and degree of organ dysfunction/failure developed by the patient either before or after ICU admission [21, 42, 43, 45], other factors have been demonstrated to play an important role, such as the place of acquisition (nosocomial vs. community-acquired infection) [42, 46] and the characteristics of the infection (site of infection, microorganism(s) involved, or extension of the infection) [47, 48]. Consequently, to reduce the evaluation of patients with severe infection and sepsis to the evaluation, quantification, and time-course pattern of MODS is a reductionist approach that will certainly overlook important information, even if it carries some prognostic accuracy [21, 49, 50].

In a general outcome prediction model, factors present at hospital admission (in other words, predisposition) are responsible for 45.9% of the explanatory power of the model

[51], and this value is also high (44.8%) in the model developed for severe infection and sepsis (SAPS 3) [36]. Although the sampling space of both models is different, which prevents definitive comparisons between them [52], the exclusive use of physiological variables in this context does not seem to be wise, since their explanatory power is low in both models (27.4% in the general model and 35.3% in the sepsis model).

For these reasons, we believe that future models should be based on the SAPS-PIRO approach, complemented by:

(a) A better distinction between risk factors for progression of the infection and for death (which we know from the work of Corinne Alberti and the European Sepsis Group to be distinct and can be modeled [48])
(b) A better distinction between general risk factors and specific risk factors for specific infections
(c) The incorporation of biomarkers (or panels of biomarkers) to evaluate the response
(d) An increase in the follow-up time of the course of organ dysfunction/failure, allowing a better follow-up of the evolution of the patient

This approach will allow the clinician to have an earlier evaluation of risk (which could drive the use of preventive or preemptive therapies), the use of specific therapies directed at the insult and at the pattern of response, and finally a better use of organ replacement therapies in patients with severe infection, sepsis, and septic shock.

References

1. Sibbald WJ, Vincent J-L. Round table conference on clinical trials for the treatment of sepsis. Brussels, March 12–14, 1994. Intensive Care Med 1995; 21:184–9
2. Jencks SF, Williams DK, Kay TL. Assessing hospital-associated deaths from discharge data. The role of length of stay and comorbidities. JAMA 1988; 260:2240–6
3. Panacek EA, Marshall JC, Albertson TE, Johnson DH, Johnson S, MacArthur RD, Miller M, Barchuk WT, Fischkoff S, Kaul M, Teoh L, Van Meter L, Daum L, Lemeshow S, Hicklin G, Doig C. Monoclonal anti-TNF: a randomized controlled sepsis study investigators. Efficacy and safety of the monoclonal anti-tumor necrosis factor antibody F(ab')2 fragment afelimomab in patients with severe sepsis and elevated interleukin-6 levels. Crit Care Med 2004; 32:2173–82
4. Cohen J, Guyatt G, Bernard GR, Calandra T, Cook D, Elbourne D, Marshall J, Nunn A, Opal S. On behalf of a UK Medical Research Council International Working Party. New strategies for clinical trials in patients with sepsis and septic shock. Crit Care Med 2001; 29:880–6
5. Bernard GR, Vincent J-L, Laterre P-F, LaRosa SP, Dhainaut J-F, Lopez-Rodriguez A, Steingrub JS, Garber GE, Helterbrand JD, Ely EW, Fisher Jr. CD. For the recombinant human activated protein C Worldwide Evaluation in Severe Sepsis (PROWESS) Study Group. Efficacy and safety of recombinant human activated protein C for severe sepsis. N Engl J Med 2001; 344: 699–709
6. Ely EW, Laterre P-F, Angus DC, Helterbrand JD, Levy H, Dhainaut J-F, Vincent J-L, Macias WL, Bernard GR. For the PROWESS Investigators. Drotrecogin alfa (activated) administration across clinically important subgroups of patients with severe sepsis. Crit Care Med 2003; 31:12–9
7. Abraham E, Laterre P-F, Garg R, Levy H, Talwar D, Trzaskoma BL, François B, Guy JS, Brückmann M, Rea-Neto A, Rossaint R, Perrotin D, Sablotzki A, Arkins N, Utterback BG,

Macias WB. For the Administration of Drotrecogin Alfa (Activated) in Early Stage Severe Sepsis (ADDRESS) Study Group. Drotrecogin Alfa (Activated) for adults with severe sepsis and a low risk of death. N Engl J Med 2005; 353:1332–41
8. Bertolini G, Rossi C, Anghileri A, Livigni S, Addis A, Poole D. Use of Drotrecogin alfa (activated) in Italian intensive care units: the results of a nationwide survey. Intensive Care Med 2007; 33:426–34
9. Kanji S, Perreault MM, Chant C, Williamson D, Burry L. Evaluating the use of Drotrecogin alfa (activated) in adult severe sepsis: a Canadian multicenter observational study. Intensive Care Med 2007; 33:517–23
10. Eichacker PQ, Natanson C. Increasing evidence that the risks of rhAPC may outweigh its benefits. Intensive Care Med 2007; 33:396–9
11. Finfer S, Marco Ranieri V, Thompson BT, Barie PS, Dhainaut J-F, Douglas IS, Gardlund B, Marshall JC, Rhodes A. Design, conduct, analysis and reporting of a multi-national placebo-controlled trial of activated protein C for persistent septic shock. Intensive Care Med 2008 (DOI 10.1007/s00134-008-1266-6)
12. Sprung CL, Annane D, Keh D, Moreno R, Singer M, Freivogel K, Weiss YG, Benbenishty J, Kalenka A, Forst H, Laterre P-F, Reinhart K, Cuthbertson BH, Payen D, Briegel J. For the CORTICUS Study Group. Hydrocortisone therapy for patients with septic shock. N Engl J Med 2008; 358:111–24
13. Annane D, Sébille V, Charpentier C, Bollaert PE, François B, Korach J-M, Capellier G, Cohen Y, Azoulay E, Troché G, Chaumet-Riffaut P, Bellissant E. Effect of treatment with low doses of hydrocortisone and fludrocortisone on mortality in patients with septic shock. JAMA 2002; 288:862–71
14. Moreno R, Sprung C, Annane D, Keh D, Singer M, Briegel J, Freivogel K, Weiss Y, Benbenishty J, Kalenka A, Forst H, Laterre P, Reinhart K, Cuthberson B, Payen D. Organ dysfunction/failure in patients with septic shock: results of the CORTICUS study [Abstract]. Intensive Care Med 2007; 33:S186
15. Petros AJ, Marshall JC, van-Saene HK. Should morbidity replace mortality as an endpoint for clinical trials in intensive care? Lancet 1995; 345:369–71
16. Knaus WA, Wagner DP, Harrell FE, Draper EA. What determines prognosis in sepsis? Evidence for a comprehensive individual patient risk assessment approach to the design and analysis of clinical trials. In: Reinhart K, Eyrich K, Sprung C, eds. Sepsis. Current Perspectives in Pathophysiology and Therapy. Springer, Berlin, 1994:23–37. (Vincent J-L, ed. Update in Intensive Care and Emergency Medicine; vol. 18)
17. Le Gall J-R, Lemeshow S, Leleu G, Klar J, Huillard J, Rué M, Teres D, Artigas A. Customized probability models for early severe sepsis in adult intensive care patients. JAMA 1995; 273:644–50
18. Knaus WA, Harrell FE, Fisher CJ, Wagner DP, Opal SM, Sadoff JC, Draper EA, Walawander CA, Conboy K, Grasela TH. The clinical evaluation of new drugs for sepsis. A prospective study design based on survival analysis. JAMA 1993; 270:1233–41
19. Knaus WA. Principles of severity stratification and outcome prediction in sepsis and shock. Intensive Care Med 1994; 20:S115
20. Vincent J-L, Moreno R, Takala J, Willats S, De Mendonça A, Bruining H, Reinhart CK, Suter PM, Thijs LG. The SOFA (sepsis-related organ failure assessment) score to describe organ dysfunction/failure. Intensive Care Med 1996; 22:707–10
21. Moreno R, Vincent J-L, Matos R, Mendonça A, Cantraine F, Thijs L, Takala J, Sprung C, Antonelli M, Bruining H, Willatts S, on behalf of the Working Group on "Sepsis-related problems" of the European Society of Intensive Care Medicine. The use of maximum SOFA score to quantify organ dysfunction/failure in intensive care. Results of a prospective, multicentre study. Intensive Care Med 1999; 25:686–96
22. Marshall JC, Cook DA, Christou NV, Bernard GR, Sprung CL, Sibbald WJ. Multiple organ dysfunction score: a reliable descriptor of a complex clinical outcome. Crit Care Med 1995; 23:1638–52

23. Le Gall JR, Klar J, Lemeshow S, Saulnier F, Alberti C, Artigas A, Teres D, The ICU scoring group. The logistic organ dysfunction system. A new way to assess organ dysfunction in the intensive care unit. JAMA 1996; 276:802–10
24. Moreno R, Pereira E, Matos R, Fevereiro T. The evaluation of cardiovascular dysfunction/failure in multiple organ failure [abstract]. Intensive Care Med 1997; 23:S153
25. Chang RW, Jacobs S, Lee B. Predicting outcome among intensive care unit patients using computerised trend analysis of daily Apache II scores corrected for organ system failure. Intensive Care Med 1988; 14:558–66
26. Timsit JF, Fosse JP, Troche G, De Lassence A, Alberti C, Garrouste-Orgeas M, Azoulay E, Chevret S, Moine P, Cohen Y. Accuracy of a composite score using daily SAPS II and LOD scores for predicting hospital mortality in ICU patients hospitalized for more than 72 h. Intensive Care Med 2001; 27:1012–21
27. Vincent JL. Dear SIRS, I'm sorry to say that I don't like you… Crit Care Med 1997; 25:372–4
28. Levy MM, Fink MP, Marshall JC, Abraham E, Angus D, Cook D, Cohen J, Opal SM, Vincent JL, Ramsay G, International Sepsis Definitions Conference. 2001 SCCM/ESICM/ACCP/ATS/SIS International Sepsis Definitions Conference. Intensive Care Med 2003; 29:530–8
29. Marshall JC, Vincent J-L, Fink MP, Cook DJ, Rubenfeld G, Foster D, Fisher Jr CJ, Faist E, Reinhart K. Measures, markers, and mediators: Toward a staging system for clinical sepsis. A Report of the Fifth Toronto Sepsis Roundtable, Toronto, Ontario, Canada, October 25–26, 2000. Crit Care Med 2003; 31:1560–7
30. Vincent J-L, Wendon J, Groeneveld J, Marshall JC, Streat S, Carlet J. The PIRO Concept: O is for organ dysfunction. Crit Care 2003; 7:260–4
31. Angus DC, Burgner D, Wunderink R, Mira JP, Gerlach H, Wiedermann CJ, Vincent J-L. The PIRO Concept: P is for predisposition. Crit Care 2003; 7:248–51
32. Gerlach H, Dhainaut JF, Harbarth S, Reinhart K, Marshall JC, Levy M. The PIRO Concept: R is for response. Crit Care 2003; 7:256–9
33. Vincent J-L, Opal S, Torres A, Bonten M, Cohen J, Wunderink R. The PIRO Concept: I is for infection. Crit Care 2003; 7:252–5
34. Finkielman JD, Dara SI, Mohammad Z, Sujay B, Afessa B. Sepsis mortality prediction based on predisposition, infection, response and organ dysfunction (PIRO) [Abstract]. Crit Care Med 2004; 32:A134
35. Metnitz PG, Moreno RP, Almeida E, Jordan B, Bauer P, Campos RA, Iapichino G, Edbrooke D, Capuzzo M, Le Gall JR, SAPS 3 Investigators. SAPS 3. From evaluation of the patient to evaluation of the intensive care unit. Part 1: Objectives, methods and cohort description. Intensive Care Med 2005; 31:1336–44
36. Moreno RP, Metnitz B, Adler L, Hoechtl A, Bauer P, Metnitz PGH, SAPS 3 Investigators. Sepsis mortality prediction based on predisposition, infection and response. Intensive Care Med 2008; 34:496–504
37. Lisboa T, Diaz E, Sa-Borges M, Socias A, Sole-Violan J, Rodríguez A, Rello J. The ventilator-associated pneumonia PIRO Score: a tool for predicting ICU mortality and health-care resources use in ventilator-associated pneumonia. Chest 2008; 134:1208–16
38. Rello J, Rodriguez A, Lisboa T, Gallego M, Lujan M, Wunderink R. PIRO score for community-acquired pneumonia: A new prediction rule for assessment of severity in intensive care unit patients with community-acquired pneumonia. Crit Care Med 2009; 37:456–462
39. Flaatten H. Epidemiology of sepsis in Norway in 1999. Crit Care 2004; 8:R180–R4
40. Martin GS, Mannino DM, Eaton S, Moss M. The epidemiology of sepsis in the United States from 1979 through 2000. N Engl J Med 2003; 348:1546–54
41. Harrison DA. The epidemiology of severe sepsis in England, Wales and Northern Ireland, 1996 to 2004: secondary analysis of a high quality clinical database, the ICNARC Case Mix Programme Database. Crit Care 2006; 10:R42

42. Martin CM, Priestap F, Fisher H, Fowler RA, Heyland DK, Keenan SP, Longo CJ, Morrison T, Bentley D, Antman N. For the STAR registry investigators. A prospective, observational registry of patients with severe sepsis: The Canadian Sepsis Treatment And Response Registry. Crit Care Med 2008; 10.1097/CCM.0b013e31819285f0
43. Dellinger RP, Levy MM, Carlet JM, Bion J, Parker MM, Jaeschke R, Reinhart K, Angus DC, Brun-Buisson C, Beale R, Calandra T, Dhainaut J-F, Gerlach H, Harvey M, Marini JJ, Marshall J, Ranieri M, Ramsay G, Sevransky J, Thompson BT, Townsend S, Vender JS, Zimmerman JL, Vincent J-L. Surviving Sepsis Campaign: International guidelines for management of severe sepsis and septic shock: 2008. Intensive Care Med 2008; 34:17–60
44. Rangel-Frausto MS, Pittet D, Costigan M, Hwang T, Davis CS, Wenzel RP. The natural history of the systemic inflammatory response syndrome (SIRS). A prospective study. JAMA 1995; 273:117–23
45. Alberti C, Brun-Buisson C, Goodman SV, Guidici D, Granton J, Moreno R, Smithies M, Thomas O, Artigas A, Le Gall J-R. Influence of systemic inflammatory response syndrome and sepsis on outcome of critically ill infected patients. Am J Respir Crit Care Med 2003; 168:77–84
46. Alberti C, Brun-Buisson C, Burchardi H, Martin C, Goodman S, Artigas A, Sicignano A, Palazzo M, Moreno R, Boulmé R, Lepage E, Le Gall J-R. Epidemiology of sepsis and infection in ICU patients from an international multicentre cohort study. Intensive Care Med 2002; 28:108–21
47. Rangel-Frausto MS. The epidemiology of bacterial sepsis. Infect Clin N Am 1999; 13: 299–312
48. Alberti C, Brun-Buisson C, Chevret S, Antonelli M, Goodman SV, Martin C, Moreno R, Ochagavia AR, Palazzo M, Werdan K, Le Gall JR, for the European Sepsis Study. Systemic inflammatory response and progression to severe sepsis in critically ill infected patients. Am J Respir Crit Care Med 2005; 171:461–8
49. Ferreira FL, Bota DP, Bross A, Mélot C, Vincent JL. Serial evaluation of the SOFA score to predict outcome in critically ill patients. JAMA 2001; 286:1754–8
50. Clermont G, Kaplan V, Moreno R, Vincent JL, Linde-Zwirble WT, Van Hout B, Angus DC. Dynamic microsimulation to model multiple outcomes in cohorts of critically ill patients. Intensive Care Med 2004; 30:2237–44
51. Moreno RP, Metnitz PG, Almeida E, Jordan B, Bauer P, Campos RA, Iapichino G, Edbrooke D, Capuzzo M, Le Gall JR, SAPS 3 Investigators. SAPS 3. From evaluation of the patient to evaluation of the intensive care unit. Part 2: Development of a prognostic model for hospital mortality at ICU admission. Intensive Care Med 2005; 31:1345–55
52. Moreno R, Jordan B, Metnitz P. The changing prognostic determinants in the critically ill patient. In: Vincent JL, ed. 2007 Yearbook of Intensive Care and Emergency Medicine. Springer, Berlin, 2007:899–907

Community-Acquired Pneumonia Management Based on the PIRO System. A New Therapeutic Paradigm

Ignacio Martin-Loeches and Jordi Rello

In 2001, an International Sepsis Definition Conference [1] agreed to assess the strengths and weaknesses of the criteria for sepsis established in 1991 [2], and, if necessary, to update them. The update was necessary because the current understanding of host response was very simplistic, and the concepts of sepsis, severe sepsis, and septic shock were very robust for daily clinical practice. Moreover, the signs and symptoms of sepsis are more varied than the initial criteria. A staging system had to be developed that would characterize the progression of sepsis. A new system was proposed based on four features – predisposition, infection, response, and organ dysfunction – the PIRO system [3–6].

This new conceptual framework for understanding sepsis, called the PIRO concept, is a classification scheme that can stratify patients based on their predisposing conditions, the nature and extend of the insult, the nature and magnitude of the host response, and the degree of the concomitant organ dysfunction. Conceptually, it was modeled on the TNM classification, which has been successfully used to define prognostic indicators in clinical oncology. PIRO was introduced as a hypothesis-generating model for future research, but its practical applications were limited. In this chapter we propose a new paradigm for the management of CAP based on the PIRO system (Table 1).

1
Predisposition

1.1
Aging

Elderly patients are more susceptible to pneumonia than younger populations. The key of success among this group of patients is based on prevention.

Several studies have documented the clinical and economic effects of influenza vaccination. Influenza vaccination programs can reduce hospitalizations and mortality in the

---

J. Rello (✉)
Critical Care Department, Joan XXIII University Hospital, University Rovira i Virgili, IISPV, CIBER Enfermedades Respiratorias (CIBERes) Tarragona, Spain
e-mail: jrello.hj23.ics@gencat.cat

Table 1 Community-acquired pneumonia management based on the PIRO system: a new therapeutic paradigm

Predisposition	Response	Insult	Organ dysfunction
1. Aging	1. Hypoxemia	1. Antibiotics	1. Early-goal directed therapy
2. Immuno-deficiencies	2. Neutropenia	2. Targeting bacterial virulence	
	3. Glucose control		2. Noninvasive mechanical ventilation
3. Genetic factors	4. Corticosteroids	3. Bacteremia	
4. Smoking cessation	5. Macrolides	3.1. Combination 3.2. Immuno-globulins	3. Low tidal volume ventilatory strategy
5. COPD	6. Activated protein C (DrotAA)	4. Multilobar pneumonia	4. Continuous hemodiafiltration
		5. Surgical drainage for empyema	

elderly, and are therefore cost-effective strategies to implement. Studies have documented a 30–50% reduction in hospitalization and a decrease in mortality [7].

The pneumococcal vaccine currently in use is designed to elicit protective antibodies against 23 of 83 known capsular serotypes of *S. pneumoniae*. These serotypes cause 90% of the invasive pneumococcal diseases and include most penicillin-resistant strains [8].

There is significant evidence that malnutrition is a risk factor for pneumonia in older patients [9]. However, evaluating the benefits of nutritional intervention and vitamin supplementation is difficult and their role as a preventive strategy remains uncertain.

1.2
Immunodeficiencies

Immunization against influenza and increasingly resistant pneumococci can play a critical role in the prevention of pneumonia. Patients who are immunosuppressed due to chronic disease or treatment may not present sustained titers of protective antibodies and should be considered for revaccination after 6 years [10].

1.3
Genetic Factors

Despite substantial advances in our understanding of the biology of pneumonia, improvements in clinical outcomes have been more sporadic and, with a few notable exceptions, are due to improvements in supportive care rather than to specific therapies. As a result, morbidity, mortality, and cost remain high. Research into the genetic determinants and the assessment of the clinical importance of genetic variation is often neglected or underestimated. While it is clear that gene sequencing and manipulation of experimental models have provided insight into the biology of the inflammatory response to infection, these technologies and their application to the study of naturally occurring human genetic variation have yet to provide the same insight or clinical benefit.

Variations in genes encoding important components of the inflammatory response and the microbial recognition system are likely to be involved in the development of pneumonia. These molecules include tumor necrosis factor (TNF), the interleukin-1 (IL-1) family, IL-10, and angiotensin-converting enzyme, as well as others that play important roles in antigen recognition, such as the mannose-binding lectin, CD-14, and toll-like receptors [11].

Most genetic traits associated with severe infection are related to defects in innate immune responses. Some, such as complement deficiencies, have been recognized for some time, while other more recently described traits are neutrophil defects, alterations in pattern recognition molecules, such as CD14 and TLRs, and variations in cytokine expression [12].

Genetic epidemiologic studies suggest a strong genetic influence on the outcome of CAP, and genetics may explain the wide variation in the individual response to infection that has long puzzled clinicians. Novel therapeutic strategies are currently being developed in experimental models to modulate the inflammatory response in the host.

1.4
Smoking Cessation

Smoking is the main risk factor in the development of chronic obstructive pulmonary disease (COPD), which is characterized by chronic respiratory symptoms and airway obstruction [13]. Pathological changes in the lungs include: increased inflammation, fibrosis of the airway wall, and destruction of alveolar attachments. Until now, smoking cessation has been the only treatment effective in slowing the rapid decline in forced expiratory volume in 1 s (FEV_1) and therefore curbing the progression of the disease. Moreover, smoking cessation halves the risk of suffering from CAP in the following 5 years [14].

1.5
Chronic Obstructive Pulmonary Disease

COPD patients are frequently admitted to hospital for CAP and a severe progression is not uncommon among this subgroup of patient. This high incidence appears to be due to altered pulmonary defense mechanisms. Moreover, as our group reported elsewhere, this selected population of patients has a greater need for mechanical ventilation [15].

Another controversial issue is the use of inhaled corticosteroids (ICS) in stable COPD patients, as it has been reported in a recent meta-analysis. ICS therapy does not affect 1-year all-cause mortality, but is associated with a higher risk of pneumonia. Future studies should determine whether specific subsets of patients with COPD benefit from ICS therapy [16].

COPD patients should be given annual influenza vaccinations, because viral infections may predispose to acute exacerbations of COPD. The resolution of the exacerbation could lead to residual bronchiolitis and bronchiectasis. Moreover, in a recent study of a large series of nonresponding CAP patients. Menendez et al. [17] found that influenza vaccination, the administration of antibiotics, and COPD were protective factors for nonresponse to initial antibiotics.

2
Insult

2.1
Antibiotics

The most important point in therapy is to eradicate the infecting organism, with the resulting resolution of the clinical disease. Appropriate antibiotic should be chosen according to the causative microorganism and its susceptibility. Although CAP can be caused by different pathogens, *S. pneumoniae* remains the leading bacterium in all groups of patients [18], followed by *H. influenzae* and *L. pneumophila*. Other bacteria should be considered in particular host subgroups. For older outpatients and those with comorbid illness such as COPD, aerobic Gram-negative bacilli including *P. aeruginosa* are increasingly common causes of pneumonia in the community [19]. Recently, methicillin-resistant *S. aureus* (MRSA) has emerged as a cause of severe pulmonary infections. *S. aureus, M. catarrhalis, M. tuberculosis*, and endemic fungi must also be considered, especially in compromised hosts [20].

S. pneumoniae is the most frequent microorganism in severe CAP. Increasing pneumococcal antibiotic resistance has led physicians to shift from penicillin to broader spectrum β-lactams, such as third-generation cephalosporins, as first choice for empi-rical therapy. The ability to cover penicillin-resistant pneumococci at the same time as atypical pathogens with the newer quinolones has also contributed to their increasing popularity.

Prompt initiation of antimicrobial therapy is crucial for optimizing survival in patients with CAP, and the first antibiotic dose seems to be pivotal for optimizing the odds of survival. Meehan et al. [21] found that initiating antibiotics in the first 8 h was associated with improved 30-day survival in elderly patients after adjustment for risk stratification and other processes of care. Also among elderly patients with CAP, Kahn et al. [22] found a decreased 30-day mortality in patients in whom antibiotics were administered in within 4 h (or within 2 h for immunocompromised patients). Although this study adjusted for sickness at admission, it did not adjust for other processes of care. A study using Medicare data of 13,771 patients revealed that antibiotic administration within 4 h after arrival to the hospital significantly reduced mortality from 7.4 to 6.8% [23]. Waterer et al. also observed better outcomes in patients with CAP when antibiotics were administered within 4 h [24].

2.2
Targeting Bacterial Virulence

A number of bacterial surface constituents and secreted products contribute to the severity of infections. Enzymes such as hemolysins, streptolysins, nucleases, proteases, lipases, and hyaluronidase convert host tissues into nutrients for bacterial growth. Surface proteins also help bacteria evade the immune system by preventing opsonization and phagocytosis by the polymorphonuclear leukocytes. In addition, some bacteria produce exotoxins, also known as superantigens, which are potent inducers of the host immune system.

Because antibacterial agents differ in their ability to attenuate virulence factors independent of bacterial spectrum, substantial effort has been directed toward defining the antivirulence pharmacology of various antibacterial agents. The rapid bactericidal activity of cell-wall active agents such as penicillin against virulent pathogens may lead to increased release of bacterial endotoxins and exotoxins.

There is a need to focus on treatment modalities that may reduce production of exotoxins as well as eradicate bacteria in order to decrease the overall morbidity and mortality associated with severe infections. The protein synthesis inhibitor clindamycin is frequently administered for treatment of severe infections – especially necrotizing fasciitis – due to its ability to inhibit exotoxin production. Numerous in vitro and in vivo studies have investigated that this enhanced efficacy of clindamycin could be related to several inherent properties, such as activity unaffected by inoculum size or stage of growth, a long postantibiotic effect, and inhibition of *S. pyogenes* virulence factors, particularly M protein [25]. Although clindamycin has no activity against Gram-negative organisms, its ability to decrease production of endotoxin has been investigated showing that pretreatment with clindamycin significantly decreased mortality and cytokine (TNF-α, IL-1β) production.

2.3
Bacteremia

Bacteremia has been traditionally associated with poor outcomes in patients with CAP [26]. After the introduction of antibiotic therapy, the mortality rate has been dramatically reduced to 17% n adults with pneumococcal bacteremic CAP treated with penicillin [27]. The case-fatality rate in bacteremic pneumococcal disease has also been shown to differ up to fourfold (5–20%) depending on the country, which may in part be explained by differences in disease severity and in the underlying conditions in the populations studied. Interestingly, the CAPO group [28] reported that pneumococcal bacteremia does not increase the risk of poor outcomes in patients with CAP. Moreover, invasive pneumococcal pneumonia management can be based on combination therapy and the use of immunoglobulins.

2.3.1
Combination

In patients with bacteremic pneumococcal illness, several authors [29–31] have associated combination antibiotic therapy with lower mortality among critically ill patients.

Combination with a macrolide and β-lactam agent for treatment of bacteremic pneumococcal pneumonia has several potential mechanisms [32] that may explain this effect: antimicrobial synergism, differences in the kill rates of pathogens, antimicrobial tolerance, the effect of macrolides [33] on cytokine production or adherence by pneumococci to respiratory epithelial cells [34], and the coexistence of atypical pathogens. Among these possibilities, we believe that the possible coexistence of atypical pathogens and the immunomodulating effect of the macrolides are the most plausible.

2.3.2
Immunoglobulins

Animal studies have reported that the use of intravenous immunoglobulins (IVIG) was effective against *S. pneumoniae* invasive pneumonia [35]. Moreover, IVIG, which contains various immunoglobulin G antibodies, may have a role in the treatment of invasive infections. IVIG [36] has been used for the treatment of patients with Panton-Valentine leukocidin-associated staphylococcal pneumonia [37]. The use of passive immunotherapy [38] is also being developed, but its potential benefit remains unclear in CAP and further investigation is warranted.

2.4
Multilobar Pneumonia

Chest X-rays are the cornerstone of the diagnosis of pneumonia in clinical studies and depict part of the insult due to increased consolidation or immunological injury to the lung after the infection. However, their role as a prognostic tool is much less clear. While multilobar infiltrates have been associated with a worse prognosis in patients with CAP, only the presence of pleural effusions is included in the widely used pneumonia severity index and none at all are used in the CURB-65. Although it is not uncommon in clinical practice to repeat the chest X-ray within 24–48 h of admission to the ICU in patients with CAP, there are very few data on the clinical relevance of changes in radiological images in these patients during this time frame. While deterioration in the chest X-ray may be expected to be associated with a higher risk of adverse outcome, exploring this hypothesis, Lisboa et al. [39] found that an increase in pulmonary infiltrates of more than 50% in the first 48 h is a significant adverse prognostic sign which more than trebled the risk of death. Given the persistently high mortality rate reported for patients with CAP admitted to the ICU, the identification of subgroups of patients at higher risk who may benefit from targeted interventions is a significant step forward.

2.5
Surgical Drainage for Empyema

Empyema most commonly occurs in the setting of bacterial pneumonia. Between 20 and 60% of all cases of pneumonia are associated with parapneumonic effusion Mortality related to empyema is associated with respiratory failure and systemic sepsis, which occurs when the immune response and antibiotics are unable to control the infection [40]. Drainage is performed to remove the collection and to improve outcomes. The proper intervention depends on the severity of the disease and ranges from minimally invasive catheter drainage to open surgical decortication. In 2000, the American College of Chest Physicians [41] reviewed the literature and issued a consensus statement on the medical and surgical treatment of parapneumonic effusions. In the setting of a parapneumonic effusion, the following findings suggest a moderate or high risk for a poor outcome: large, free-flowing effusion (at least half of a hemithorax); loculated effusion or effusion with thickened parietal pleura; positive cultures or Gram stains; pleural pus; and pH < 7.20. When these findings are present, drainage is recommended. Prompt diagnosis and intervention reduce patient mortality, and delaying diagnosis or intervention could worsen the clinical course.

3
Response

3.1
Hypoxemia

Early assessment of hypoxemia may lead to a better outcome after CAP is established and can determine which subgroup of patients may benefit from intensive care management within critical care premises. While this will intuitively make sense to clinicians, information on the issue is very limited.

Current guidelines on CAP recommend oxygenation assessment (either pulse oximetry monitoring or blood gas analysis) within the first 24 h as a quality indicator This recommendation is based on expert opinion, because no evidence exists to support any particular time frame for oxygenation assessment. Blot et al. [42] reported that a delay in oxygenation assessment of less than 3 h was associated with a twofold increase in the risk of death. These findings show that the classic 24-h target for either pulse oximetry monitoring or blood gas sampling can no longer be supported in patients presenting with severe CAP to the emergency room. Based on these observations, oxygenation assessment should be performed soon after arrival at the emergency department in patients suspected of having pneumonia. Moreover, not only does early oxygenation assessment represent better outcomes on its own, but postponing oxygenation assessment for more than 1 h was also associated with a significantly longer time until initiation of antibiotic therapy.

3.2
Neutropenia

Immunoparalysis has recently been included in the pathophysiology of impaired response during the infection and worse progression. Granulocyte colony-stimulating factor (G-CSF) is an important factor in neutropoiesis. The theoretical ability of G-CSF to improve the functions [43] of both neutrophils and monocytes/macrophages provides a rationale for G-CSF therapy in non-neutropenic critically ill patients with infection [44]. A meta-analysis on the effectiveness of G-CSF has been published recently [45] as an adjunct to antimicrobials for the treatment of non-neutropenic adults with pneumonia. Cumulative data from randomized clinical trials demonstrated no difference between patients with CAP who received G-CSF and placebo regarding 28-day all-cause mortality. Therefore, the currently available information does not support the routine use of G-CSF in non-neutropenic patients with CAP.

3.3
Glucose Control

Many researchers have reported an association between hyperglycemia and adverse clinical outcomes. In 2001, Van den Berghe et al. [46] reported that in-hospital mortality in critically ill surgical patients had fallen by 33% and showed that titrating insulin infusion during intensive care to strict normoglycemia (below 110 mg dL^{-1}) strikingly reduced mortality when compared with the conventional insulin treatment on non-diabetic ICU patients that aimed for a much lower level of blood glucose. Moreover, hyperglycemia promotes complications such as critical illness polyneuropathy, bacteremia, and acute renal failure. These results were confirmed by Krinsley [47] in a mixed medical–surgical intensive care population.

To confirm the results of earlier studies and to better evaluate the impact of tight blood glucose control in a mixed ICU population, Preiser et al. [48] conducted the Glucontrol study, which found that the incidence of severe hypoglycemia (defined as a blood glucose of <40 mg dL^{-1}) was significantly more frequent in patients assigned to tighter blood glucose control. Specifically, severe hypoglycemia occurred in 8.6% of this group compared with only 2.4% ($p < 0.001$) in the less strictly controlled group. Multivariate analysis confirmed that aggressive blood glucose targets significantly increased the risk of hypoglycemia. However, there was no difference in all-cause mortality (17% vs. 15%, p = NS) between groups and the risk of death was not increased in patients who experienced severe hypoglycemia. In addition, there was no difference in length of stay between the groups. Tight blood glucose control with a target range of 80–110 mg dL^{-1} offered no apparent benefits, but increased the risk of hypoglycemia.

Investigating the value of subcutaneous insulin-by-glucose sliding scales for the management of hospitalized patients with pneumonia, Becker et al. [49] argued against their use in CAP patients.

It may be that either the target of 80–110 mg dL^{-1} is too strict or that we have insufficient tools for accurately monitoring and predicting hypoglycemia. In any event, prior approaches in which the blood glucose was allowed to drift above 200 mg dL^{-1} do not seem acceptable either. The question is not how liberal one should be in tolerating blood glucose elevation, but how one can best maximize benefit while minimizing harm.

3.4
Corticosteroids

With the concept of critical illness-related corticosteroid insufficiency (CIRI) [50] and the results of clinical trials showing respiratory immune and hemodynamic benefits, corticosteroids have reemerged as promising adjuncts for the treatment of severe sepsis. Several recent studies have tried to elucidate the pulmonary and systemic inflammatory response and have provided data on the adrenal function of patients with severe CAP [51]. In addition, the administration of systemic corticosteroids has been shown to block several arms of the inflammatory cascade [52]. The regulation of nuclear transcriptional factors can activate the gene expression of genes involved in the inflammatory response. During severe CAP, a systematic inflammation can occur; however, systemic steroids might modulate this exuberant inflammatory response. Thus, recent guidelines for the management of CAP suggest the benefit of systemic corticosteroids for patients with a severe presentation. However, the four randomized controlled trials [53–56] had a small sample size. Only in one trial [53] was the adrenal function assessed before initiation of treatment. The results showed a reduction in mortality, suggesting that the administration of corticosteroids might be beneficial in terms of survival.

However, the results of CORTICUS [57] do not support the use of corticosteroids for patients with septic shock, because they show only a beneficial effect of the stress doses of corticosteroids on the time interval to shock reversal and not on mortality, potentially explained by an increased risk of superinfection. The mortality in the placebo arm was relatively low, lower than in earlier randomized studies that stressed that doses of corticosteroids had a favorable hemodynamic effect and conferred a survival benefit in septic shock.

In view of this controversy, additional studies are needed in order to identify more clearly the patient group most likely to benefit from this therapy.

3.5
Macrolides

Antibiotic therapy has been reported to increase the outcome in septic shock patients with CAP. The study by Rodriguez et al. [58] found no difference in mortality rate between single and combination antibiotic therapy overall; however, for patients with shock, combination therapy with macrolides was associated with a survival advantage compared with single antibiotic therapy. This effect was not found in combination therapy involving quinolones. Another study, published by Restrepo et al. [59], associated the use of macrolides with decreased mortality at 30 days (hazard ratio [HR] 0.3, 95% confidence interval [CI] 0.2–0.7) and at 90 days (HR 0.3, 95% CI 0.2–0.6) in patients with severe sepsis and even in patients with macrolide-resistant pathogens (HR 0.1, 95% CI 0.02–0.5). The addition of macrolides may have benefits for severely ill patients other than only antibiotic coverage. Recent studies suggest that macrolides may have beneficial effects for patients at risk of certain infections due to their immunomodulatory effects rather than due to their antimicrobial properties [60]. The spectrum of action of these antibiotics extends to the regulation of leukocyte function and production of inflammatory mediators, control of mucus hypersecretion, resolution of inflammation, and modulation of host defense mechanisms for patients with severe CAP. Proinflammatory cytokines, such as TNF-α, IL-1, IL-6, and also anti-inflammatory cytokines such as IL-10 have been modulated by macrolides.

Recent studies have gone further, suggesting that macrolides can facilitate the killing of microorganisms in acute respiratory infections through the stimulation of neutrophil activation. On long-term administration, anti-inflammatory, T-helper type 1 lymphocyte-enhancing and biofilm-thinning actions, among others, make macrolides valid therapeutic options in chronic infectious/inflammatory disorders, even for infections with microorganisms that are not completely eradicated.

3.6
Activated Protein C

Experimental studies have shown that activated protein C (APC; drotrecogin alfa, DrotAA) exerts lung-protective effects via anticoagulant and anti-inflammatory pathways. The effectiveness of APC for the treatment of patients with severe CAP was studied in a retrospective analysis of the Efficacy and Safety of Recombinant Human Activated Protein C for Severe Sepsis (PROWESS) trial. As part of this study, a subgroup analysis was conducted in patients with severe sepsis caused by CAP, with a CURB-65 (confusion, urea, respiratory rate, blood pressure, age >65 years) score of above 3, who were treated with DrotAA [61] The results showed a relative risk reduction in mortality of 28% at 28 days, and of 14% at 90 days. The survival benefit was most pronounced in severe CAP patients with *S. pneumoniae* infection and in CAP patients at high risk of death, as indicated by an APACHE II score above 25, a Pneumonia Severity Index score above 4, or CURB-65 score above 3. On the other hand, in the subgroup of patients with CAP who were not in septic shock, the use of APC as opposed to placebo was not associated with a statistical significant reduction in all-cause in-hospital mortality (relative risk 0.68, 95% CI 0.45–1.00.) These findings should be reviewed carefully because the primary limitations of this study are its post hoc definition and the fact that it was a subgroup analysis. Given that patients were not randomized by subgroups, the estimates may be skewed by confounders. What is more, a subgroup analysis may lack the statistical power to reveal differences (type II statistical error).

4
Organ Dysfunction

4.1
Early Goal-Directed Therapy

The early stages of sepsis may be accompanied by circulatory insufficiency resulting from hypovolemia, myocardial depression, increased metabolic rate, and vasoregulatory perfusion abnormalities. As a consequence, a variety of hemodynamic combinations create a systemic imbalance between tissue oxygen supply and demand, leading to global tissue hypoxia and shock. In fact, consensus guidelines now recommend early goal-directed therapy for the first 6h of sepsis resuscitation. Despite this, however, early goal-directed therapy is still not widely used in clinical practice.

Early goal-directed therapy [62] is a more specific form of therapy used for the treatment of severe sepsis and septic shock. This approach involves adjustments of cardiac preload, afterload, and contractility to balance oxygen delivery. The main points are based on the following: in the event of hypotension and/or lactate level greater than 4 mmol L^{-1}, deliver an initial minimum of 20 mL kg^{-1} of crystalloid (or colloid equivalent). Apply vasopressors for hypotension not responding to initial fluid resuscitation to maintain mean arterial pressure (MAP) at above 65 mmHg. In the event of persistent hypotension despite fluid resuscitation (septic shock) and/or lactate levels greater than 4 mmol L^{-1} (36 mg dL^{-1}): (a) achieve a central venous pressure (CVP) of more than 8 $mmHg^2$, and (b) achieve central venous oxygen saturation (ScvO2) of more than 70%.

Moreover, septic shock must be managed aggressively during emergency department triage. Lactate clearance early in the hospital course may indicate a resolution of global tissue hypoxia and is associated with a decreased mortality rate. Higher lactate clearance after 6 h of emergency department intervention is associated with improved outcome [63].

This intervention should be targeted by (ideally objective) monitored end points so that therapy may be individualized.

4.2
Noninvasive Mechanical Ventilation

In acute exacerbation of COPD, noninvasive mechanical ventilation (NIMV) is now considered the ventilation mode of choice. For treatment of acute pulmonary edema, CPAP alone is very effective. NIMV reduces the chances of endotracheal intubation in hypoxemic respiratory failure. However, its precise role in the management of patients with severe CAP remains unclear as these patients present a high risk of NIMV failure. Only one randomized clinical trial [64] has investigated the issue to date; including 56 patients with severe CAP and acute respiratory failure (refractory hypoxemia and/or hypercapnia with acidosis), it demonstrated no difference between patients with or without NIMV in terms of hospital mortality and length of hospital stay. However, a post hoc analysis revealed that in the subgroup of patients with underlying COPD, a 2-month survival benefit was seen for those who were under NIMV (89% vs. 38%, $p = 0.05$).

4.3
Low Tidal Volume Ventilatory Strategy

Traditional tidal volumes of 10–15 mL kg^{-1} result in elevated airway pressures and overdistention of the less affected lung regions, which exacerbate or perpetuate the lung injury. Ventilation with small tidal volumes and limited airway pressures can reduce ventilator-associated lung injury due to overdistention. In a person with acute lung injury (ALI)/acute respiratory distress syndrome (ARDS) requiring mechanical ventilation, the goal must be to provide adequate oxygenation without causing morbidity from oxygen toxicity, hemodynamic compromise, barotraumas, and alveolar overdistention [65, 66].

These large tidal volumes are known to cause stretch-induced lung injury and release of inflammatory mediators. They also perpetuate the cycle of inflammation and injury in people with ALI and ARDS.

There is strong evidence that mechanical ventilation, utilizing a low tidal volume, may be beneficial. The ARDS Network trial [67] recommended mechanical ventilation at 6 mL kg^{-1} ideal body weight in patients with ALI/ARDS. A common consequence of a low tidal volume ventilatory strategy is the development of hypercapnia and respiratory acidosis, known as permissive hypercapnia. As long as adequate oxygenation is achieved, hypercapnia is an acceptable adverse effect of controlled ventilation. Contraindications to permissive hypercapnia include predisposition to increased cranial pressure (intracerebral bleeding, brain tumor, fulminant hepatic failure) and hemodynamic instability. Sedation administration should not be considered a barrier to implementing a lung-protective ventilation strategy.

4.4
Continuous Hemodiafiltration

The primary goals in management of patients with acute renal failure (ARF) when sepsis is present are to optimize hemodynamic and volume status, minimize further renal injury, correct metabolic abnormalities, and permit adequate nutrition. Unfortunately, dopamine, multiple drugs, and the use of furosemide have shown a lack of benefit in "protecting" the kidneys during the sepsis and also during severe acquired pneumonia.

Renal replacement therapy (RRT) is often required to achieve these goals while awaiting renal recovery, but the optimal dose of dialysis in patients with ARF is not known. Extrapolation of the required dialysis dose from recommendations in chronic dialysis is unlikely to be appropriate because of the lack of a steady state and differences in distribution volume of urea that are intrinsic to ARF. The impact of intermittent hemodialysis (IHD) versus continuous renal replacement therapy (CRRT) on outcomes in ARF is still controversial. Despite the conceptual advantages of continuous forms of RRT, including improved hemodynamics, easier fluid removal, and flexibility with parenteral nutrition, continuous therapies exhibit some potential drawbacks such as access-related complications, bleeding, and increased manpower or financial investments when highly sophisticated treatment devices are used.

Furthermore, the ultrafiltration dose has been a matter of debate. Its benefit remains unclear and has only been shown in reducing the plasma concentration of TNF-α in animal models [68].

A randomized study using continuous venovenous hemofiltration suggested that the ultrafiltration rate of 35 or 45 mL per kg per h presented better survival in ARF than a rate of 20 mL per kg per h. Moreover, when sepsis is present, the best survival was shown with an ultrafiltration rate of 45 mL per kg per h [69, 70].

Acknowledgments Ignacio Martin-Loeches and Jordi Rello are supported by AGAUR 2005/SGR/920, CiBeRes 06/06/0036, FISS 04/1500.

References

1. Levy MM, Fink MP, Marshall JC, et al. (2003) 2001 SCCM/ESICM/ACCP/ATS/SIS International Sepsis Definitions Conference. Crit Care Med 31(4):1250–1256

2. Bone RC, Balk RA, Cerra FB, Dellinger RP, Fein AM, Knaus WA, Schein RA, Sibbald WJ (1992) Definitions for sepsis and organ failure and guidelines for the use of innovative therapies in sepsis. Chest 101:1644–1655
3. Angus DC, Burgner D, Wunderink R, et al. (2003) The PIRO concept: P is for predisposition. Crit Care 7:248–251
4. Vincent JL, Opal S, Torres A, et al. (2003) The PIRO concept: I is for infection. Crit Care 7:252–255
5. Gerlach H, Dhainaut JF, Harbarth S, et al. (2003) The PIRO concept: R is for response. Crit Care 7:256–259
6. Vincent JL, Wendon J, Groeneveld J, et al. (2003) The PIRO concept: O is for organ dysfunction. Crit Care 7:260–264
7. Nichol K, Nordin J, Nelson D, et al. (2007) Effectiveness of influenza vaccine in the community-dwelling elderly. N Engl J Med 357:1373–1381
8. Fine MJ, Smith MA, Carson CA, et al. (1994) Efficacy of pneumococcal vaccination in adults. A meta-analysis of randomized controlled trials. Arch Int Med 154:2666–2677
9. Woo J, Ho SC, Mak YT, et al. (1994) Nutritional status of elderly patients during recovery from chest infection and the role of nutritional supplementation assessed by a prospective randomized single-blind trial. Age Ageing 23:40–48
10. Centers for Disease Control and Prevention (2001) Prevention and control of influenza: recommendations of the Advisory Committee on Immunization Practices (ACIP). MMWR 50(RR-04):1–46
11. Branger J, Florquin S, Knapp S, Leemans JC, Pater JM, Speelman P, Golenbock DT, Van der Poll T (2004) Role of toll-like receptor 4 in Gram-positive and Gram-negative pneumonia in mice. Infect Immun 72:788–794
12. Waterer GW, Wunderink RG (2005) Genetic susceptibility to pneumonia. Clin Chest Med 26:29–38
13. Almirall J, Gonzalez C, Balanzo X, Bolivar I (1999). Proportion of community-acquired pneumonia cases attributable to tobacco smoking. Chest 116:692–697
14. Nuorti JP, Butler JC, Farley MM, Harrison LH, McGeer A, Kolczak MS, et al. (2000) Cigarette smoking and invasive pneumococcal disease. Active Bacterial Core Surveillance Team. N Engl J Med 342:681–689
15. Rello J, Rodriguez A, Torres A, Roig J, Sole-Violan J, Garnacho-Montero J, de la Torre MV, Sirvent JM, Bodi M (2006) Implications of COPD in patients admitted to the intensive care unit by community-acquired pneumonia. Eur Respir J 27:1210–1216
16. Drummond MB, Dasenbrook EC, Pitz MW, Murphy DJ, Fan E (2008). Inhaled corticosteroids in patients with stable chronic obstructive pulmonary disease: a systematic review and meta-analysis. JAMA 300:2407–2416
17. Menéndez R, Torres A, Zalacaín R, et al. (2004). Risk factors of treatment failure in community-acquired pneumonia: implications for disease outcome. Thorax 59:960–965
18. Ortqvist A, Hedlund J, Kalin M (2005) *Streptococcus pneumoniae*: epidemiology, risk factors, and clinical features. Semin Respir Crit Care Med 26(6):563–574
19. Rello J, Bodi M, Mariscal D, Navarro M, Díaz E, Gallego M, Valles J (2003) Microbiological testing and outcome of patients with severe community-acquired pneumonia. Chest Jan 123(1):174–180
20. Bodi M, Rodriguez A, Sole-Violan J, Gilavert MC, Garnacho J, Blanquer J, Jimenez J, de la Torre MV, Sirvent JM, Almirall J, et al. (2005): Antibiotic prescribing for community-acquired pneumonia in the intensive care unit: impact of adherence to Infectious Diseases Society of America Guidelines on survival. Clin Infect Dis 41:1709–1716
21. Meehan TP, Fine MJ, Krumholz HM, Scinto JD, Galusha DH, Mockalis JT, et al. (1997) Quality of care, process, and outcomes in elderly patients with pneumonia. JAMA 278:2080–2084

22. Kahn LK, Rogers WH, Rubenstein LV, et al. (1990) Measuring quality of care with explicit process criteria before and after implementation of the DRG-based prospective payment system. JAMA 264:1969–1973
23. Houck PM, Bratzler DW, Nsa W, Ma A, Bartlett JG (2004) Timing of antibiotic administration and outcomes for Medicare patients hospitalized with community-acquired pneumonia. Arch Int Med 164:637–644. Abstract
24. Waterer GW, Kessler LA, Wunderink RG (2006) Delayed administration of antibiotics and atypical presentation in community-acquired pneumonia. Chest 130:11–15
25. Hirata N, Hiramatsu K, Kishi K, Yamasaki T, Ichimiya T, Nasu M (2001) Pretreatment of mice with clindamycin improves survival of endotoxic shock by modulating the release of inflammatory cytokines. Antimicrob Agents Chemother 45:2638–2642
26. Tilghman C, Finland M (1937) Clinical significance of bacteremia in pneumococci pneumonia. Arch Int Med 59:602–619
27. Austrian R, Gold J (1964) Pneumococcal bacteremia with especial reference to bacteremic pneumococcal pneumonia. Ann Int Med 60:759–776
28. Bordon J, Peyrani P, Brock GN, Blasi F, Rello J, File T, Ramirez J (2008) The presence of pneumococcal bacteremia does not influence clinical outcomes in patients with community-acquired pneumonia: results from the Community-Acquired Pneumonia Organization (CAPO) International Cohort study. Chest 133:618–624
29. Waterer GW, Somes GW, Wunderick RG (2001) Monotherapy may be suboptimal for severe bacteremic pneumococcal pneumonia. Arch Intern Med 161:1837–1842
30. Mart?´nez JA, Horcajada JP, Almeda M, et al. (2003) Addition of a macrolide to a b-lactam-based empirical antibiotic regimen is associated with lower in-hospital mortality for patients with bacteremic pneumococcal pneumonia. Clin Infect Dis 36:389–395
31. Baddour LM, Yu VL, Klugman KP, Feldman C, Ortqvist A, Rello J, Morris AJ, Luna CM, Snydman DR, Ko WC, et al. (2004) Combination antibiotic therapy lowers mortality among severely ill patients with pneumococcal bacteremia. Am J Respir Crit Care Med 170:440–444
32. Yamasawa H, Osikawa O, Ohno S, Sugiyama Y (2004) Macrolides inhibit epithelial cell-mediated neutrophil survival by modulating granulocyte macrophage colony-stimulating factor release. Am J Respir Cell Mol Biol 30:569–575
33. Reato G, Cuffini AM, Tullio V, et al. (2004) Immunomodulating effect of antimicrobial agents on cytokine production by human polymorphonuclear neutrophils. Int J Antimicrob Agents 23:150–154
34. Giamarellos-Bourboulis EJ, Adamis T, Laoutaris G, et al. (2004) Immunomodulatory clarithromycin treatment of experimental sepsis and acute pyelonephritis caused by multidrug-resistant *Pseudomonas aeruginosa*. Antimicrob Agents Chemother 48:93–99
35. De Hennezel L, Ramisse F, Binder P, et al. (2001) Effective combination therapy for invasive pneumococcal pneumonia with ampicillin and intravenous immunoglobulins in a mouse model. Antimicrob Agents Chemother 45:316–318
36. Chiou CC, Yu LV (2006) Severe pneumococcal pneumonia: new strategies for management. Curr Opin Crit Care 12:470–476
37. Morgan MS (2007) Diagnosis and treatment of Panton–Valentine leukocidin (PVL)-associated staphylococcal pneumonia. Int J Antimicrob Agents 30:289–296
38. Casadevall A, Scharff M (1995) Return to the past: the case for antibody-based therapy in infectious diseases. Clin Infect Dis 21:150–161
39. Lisboa T, Blot S, Waterer GW, Canalis E, de Mendoza D, Rodriguez A, Rello J (2009) Radiological progression of pulmonary infiltrates predicts a worse prognosis in severe community-acquired pneumonia than bacteremia. Chest 135:165–172
40. Lim TK (2001) Management of parapneumonic pleural effusion. Curr Opin Pulm Med Jul 7(4):193–197
41. Colice GL, Curtis A, Deslauriers J, et al. (2000) Medical and surgical treatment of parapneumonic effusions: an evidence-based guideline. Chest 118(4):1158–1171

42. Blot SI, Rodriguez A, Solé-Violán J, Blanquer J, Almirall J, Rello J (2007) Effects of delayed oxygenation assessment on time to antibiotic delivery and mortality in patients with severe community-acquired pneumonia. Crit Care Med 35:2509–2514
43. Stephens DP, Fisher DA, Currie BJ (2002) An audit of the use of granulocyte colony-stimulating factor in septic shock. Int Med J 32:143–148
44. Hartung T (1999) Granulocyte colony-stimulating factor; its potential role in infectious disease. Acquir Immune Defic Syndr; 13 Suppl 2:3–9
45. Cheng AC, Stephens DP, Currie BJ (2007) Granulocyte-colony stimulating factor (G-CSF) as an adjunct to antibiotics in the treatment of pneumonia in adults. Cochrane Database Syst Rev; CD004400
46. Van den Berghe G, Wouters P, Weekers F, Verwaest C, Bruyninckx F, Schetz M, Vlasselaers D, Ferdinande P, Lauwers P, Bouillon R (2001) Intensive insulin therapy in critically ill patients. N Engl J Med 345:1359–1367
47. Krinsley JS (2004) Effect of an intensive glucose management protocol on the mortality of critically ill adult patients. Mayo Clin Proc 79:992–1000
48. Preiser JC (2007) Intensive glycemic control in med-surg patients (European Glucontrol trial). Program and abstracts of the Society of Critical Care Medicine 36th Critical Care Congress, February 17–21, Orlando, Florida
49. Becker T, Moldoveanu A, Cukierman T, et al, (2007) Clinical outcomes associated with the use of subcutaneous insulin-by-glucose sliding scales to manage hyperglycemia in hospitalized patients with pneumonia. Diab Res Clin Pract 78:392–397
50. Cooper MS, Stewart PM (2003) Corticosteroid Insufficiency in Acutely Ill Patients N Engl J Med 348:727–734
51. Monton C, Ewig S, Torres A, et al. (1999) Role of glucocorticoids on inflammatory response in nonimmunosuppressed patients with pneumonia: a pilot study. Eur Respir J 14:218–220
52. Barnes PJ (2006) Corticosteroid effects on cell signaling. Eur Respir J 27:413–426
53. Mikami K, Suzuki M, Kitagawa H, et al. (2007) Efficacy of corticosteroids in the treatment of community-acquired pneumonia requiring hospitalization. Lung 185:249–255
54. Confalonieri M, Urbino R, Potena A, et al. (2005) Hydrocortisone infusion in patients with severe community-acquired pneumonia: results of a randomized clinical trial. Am J Respir Crit Care Med 171:242–248
55. Marik P, Kraus P, Sribante J, et al. (1993) Hydrocortisone and tumor necrosis factor in severe community-acquired pneumonia: a randomized controlled study. Chest 104:389–392
56. Wagner HN, Bennet IL, Lasagna L, et al. (1995) The effect of hydrocortisone upon the course of pneumococcal pneumonia treated with penicillin. Bull Johns Hopkins Hosp 98:197–215
57. Sprung CL, Annane D, Keh D, Moreno R, Singer M, Freivogel K, Weiss YG, Benbenishty J, Kalenka A, Forst H, Laterre PF, Reinhart K, Cuthbertson BH, Payen D, Briegel J, CORTICUS (2008) Hydrocortisone therapy for patients with septic shock. N Engl J Med 358:111–124
58. Rodriguez A, Mendia A, Sirvent JM, Barcenilla F, de la Torre-Prados MV, Sole-Violan J, Rello J (2007) Combination antibiotic therapy improves survival in patients with community-acquired pneumonia and shock. Crit Care Med Jun 35:1493–1498
59. Restrepo MI, Mortensen EM, Waterer GW, Wunderink RG, Coalson JJ, Anzueto A (2009) Impact of macrolide therapy on mortality for patients with severe sepsis due to pneumonia Eur Respir J 33(1):153–159
60. Parnham MJ (2005) Immunomodulatory effects of antimicrobials in the therapy of respiratory tract infections. Curr Opin Infect Dis 18:125–131
61. Laterre PF, Garber G, Levy H, Wunderink R, Kinasewitz GT, Sollet JP, Maki DG, Bates B, Yan SC, Dhainaut JF (2005) Severe community-acquired pneumonia as a cause of severe sepsis: data from the PROWESS study. Crit Care Med 33:952–961

62. Rivers E, Nguyen B, Havstad S, et al. (2001) Early goal-directed therapy in the treatment of severe sepsis and septic shock. N Engl J Med 345:1368–1377
63. Nguyen HB, Rivers EP, Knoblich BP, Jacobsen G, Muzzin A, Ressler JA, Tomlanovich MC (2004) Early lactate clearance is associated with improved outcome in severe sepsis and septic shock. Crit Care Med 32:1637–1642
64. Confalonieri M, Potena A, Carbone G, et al. (1999) Acute respiratory failure in patients with severe community-acquired pneumonia. A prospective randomized evaluation of noninvasive ventilation. Am J Respir Crit Care Med 160:1585–1591
65. Dreyfuss D, Saumon G (1998) Ventilator-induced lung injury: lessons from experimental studies. Am J Respir Crit Care Med 157:294–323
66. Slutsky AS, Tremblay LN (1998) Multiple system organ failure. Is mechanical ventilation a contributing factor? Am J Respir Crit Care Med 157:1721–1725
67. The Acute Respiratory Distress Syndrome Network. (2000) Ventilation with lower tidal volumes as compared with traditional tidal volumes for acute lung injury and the acute respiratory distress syndrome. N Engl J Med 342:1301–1308
68. Rogiers P, Zhang H, Smail N, et al. (1999) Continuous venovenous hemofiltration improves cardiac performance by mechanisms other than tumor necrosis factor-alpha attenuation during endotoxic shock. Crit Care Med 27:1848–1855
69. Ronco C, Bellomo R, Homel P, et al. (2000) Effects of different doses in continuous venovenous haemofiltration on outcomes of acute renal failure: a prospective randomised trial. Lancet 356:26–30
70. Jakob SM, Frey FJ, Uehlinger DE (1996) Does continuous renal replacement therapy favourably influence the outcome of the patients? Nephrol Dial Transplant 11:1250–1255

Ventilator-Associated Pneumonia PIRO Score

4

Emili Díaz and Thiago Lisboa

1
Introduction

Ventilator-associated pneumonia (VAP) is the leading nosocomial infection of intensive care unit (ICU) acquisition with an incidence rate between 5 and 16 episodes per 1,000 ventilator-days [1], affecting the course of 8–28% of patients on mechanical ventilation [2]. VAP carries an increase in healthcare resources, and affected patients spend more time in the ICU and need to be ventilated for more days. In addition, some patients die because of this infection.

Several scores have been designed to stratify patients according to disease severity at ICU admission. Some examples are the Acute Physiology and Chronic Health Evaluation (APACHE) score, versions I, II, III, or IV, and the Simplified Acute Physiology Score (SAPS), versions I, II, or III. When patients are infected, the following scores can be used: Sequential Organ Failure Assessment (SOFA), Multiple Organ Dysfunction Score (MODS), and the Organ Dysfunction and/or Infection (ODIN) score.

Some scores are disease-specific. In this way, severe community-acquired pneumonia (CAP) patients can be classified into different risk groups using the Pneumonia Severity Index (PSI) [3], CURB-65 [4], or American Thoracic Society major and minor criteria for risk classification [5].

Scores have been found to be useful for the classification of different groups. Their utility for individuals, however, is thought to be uncertain. However, therapeutic strategies such as drotrecogin alfa (activated) have been approved for patients with severe sepsis and high severity of more than 24 as determined by the APACHE II score. Currently, the study ACCESS (A Controlled Comparison of Eritoran Tetrasodium and Placebo in Patients with Severe Sepsis) is recruiting participants, and inclusion criteria are age (18 years or older), confirmed early-onset severe sepsis, and an APACHE II score between 21 and 37 points [6].

E. Díaz (*)
Critical Care Department, Joan XXIII University Hospital, University Rovira & Virgili, Institut Pere Virgili, CIBER Enfermedades Respiratorias (CIBERES), Tarragona, Spain
e-mail: emilio.diaz.santos@gmail.com

However, no score has been developed to assess severity in patients who develop VAP at the time of diagnosis. The APACHE II score at admission has been used in matched cohort studies of VAP to compare patients with and without VAP. In a matched cohort study, patients with VAP due to methicillin-resistant *Staphylococcus aureus* (MRSA) were matched with patients without MRSA VAP [7]. Matching was based on the admission diagnosis, time at the ICU before VAP onset, and APACHE II score. The MRSA VAP patients had a higher mortality rate, which shows the inability of the APACHE II score to classify patients with VAP at the time of diagnosis. Previously, Rello et al. designed a study to assess the impact of severity of illness at different times using the Mortality Probability Models (MPM II) [8]. The authors did not observe differences in mean MPM II between survivors and nonsurvivors at the time of ICU admission, nor 24 h after admission. In contrast, differences were observed in MPM II at the time of pneumonia diagnosis [8], with the authors concluding that when pneumonia is diagnosed severity of illness is the most important predictor of survival. In addition, pneumonia by *Pseudomonas aeruginosa* increased the mortality rate.

In 1992 Bone et al. published probably one of the most relevant articles in *Critical Care Medicine* on the definitions of sepsis and organ failure and guidelines for the use of innovative therapies in sepsis [9]. This article was the state of the art and provided the final classification for sepsis and sepsis-related syndromes. When a group of experts reviewed the 1992 sepsis guidelines they found no evidence to change the definitions [10]. Moreover, the classification of sepsis, severe sepsis, and septic shock was found to be inadequate for staging septic patients. In analogy to the TNM classification system in oncology, this meeting of experts came up with the concept of PIRO. This concept, based on predisposition (P), insult/infection (I), host response (R), and organ dysfunction (O), started with the authors' idea of being able to discriminate morbidity from infection and morbidity from host response to infection. The bedside utility of this tool was poorly developed, and as stated by Moreno et al., although interesting and promising it remained conceptual [11]. Moreno and colleagues subsequently published an analysis of mortality based on a modification of the PIRO concept (predisposition, insult/infection, and host response) in the SAPS III study database [11].

2
Ventilator-Associated Pneumonia and the PIRO Concept

VAP is defined as a lower respiratory tract infection occurring in patients on mechanical ventilation for more than 48 h. Its clinical diagnosis is based on the presence on a chest roentgenogram of new or persistent opacities in concurrence with local purulent secretions from an endotracheal tube and systemic manifestation of an infection process – fever, leukocytosis, or leukopenia. VAP is the leading nosocomial infection in the ICU setting and can increase the time on a ventilator by 10 days, the time of ICU admission by 6 days, and the length of hospital stay by 11 days [1]. Associated mortality for patients with VAP ranges between 0 and more than 50% [2]. In the ICU setting, attending physicians daily have to confront patients in whom a pulmonary infection can complicate their previous critical situation. A PIRO-based model could be useful for assessing severity and stratifying mortality risk in VAP patients. How can the PIRO concept assess severity in VAP patients?

2.1
Predisposition

Premorbid conditions may predispose patients to infectious complications in the ICU. The presence of specific comorbid conditions may be associated with poorer outcomes in VAP patients.

The effect of age has been studied in ICU patients. Age is a component of major prognostic tools such as the APACHE II or SAPS III scores. In a prospective study comparing different modalities for the diagnosis and treatment of VAP, risk factors associated with clinical failure were analyzed, and death was the most common reason for clinical failure [12]. In this study four factors were found to be associated with clinical failure in patients with VAP: older age, duration of ventilation before enrolment, presence of neurologic disease at admission, and failure of the PaO_2/FiO_2 ratio to improve by day 3.

The reason for admission to the ICU is a very important factor when analyzing outcomes. Trauma has been found to be associated with better outcomes in patients developing VAP when compared with surgical [13] or medical and surgical populations [14]. In a prospective and observational study in a medical surgical ICU, Myny et al. showed that factors independently associated with death were higher SAPS II scores and reason for admission other than trauma [14].

Medical conditions predisposing patients to serious infections such as chronic obstructive pulmonary disease (COPD), immunocompromise, chronic heart failure, chronic hepatopathy, and chronic renal failure can have an impact on the severity of VAP episodes.

COPD is a disease state characterized by the presence of airflow due to chronic bronchitis or emphysema. In the United States, COPD ranks fourth as the main cause of chronic morbidity and mortality [15]. Mortality has been increasing from 1960, reaching 50 deaths/100,000 population in 1996 [16]. The total cost of COPD was calculated to be U.S. $23.9 billion in 1993, ranking second in the overall costs for lung diseases. VAP in COPD patients has been associated with an increased risk of mortality [17]. In a prospective case-control study, all COPD patients who required intubation and mechanical ventilation were matched according to time of mechanical ventilation before VAP onset, age, a SAP II score on ICU admission, and ICU admission category. Seventy-seven patients developed VAP and were successfully matched. VAP was the only factor independently associated with ICU mortality [17].

Immune system deficiency has been found to be associated with a poor prognosis for infections. Ibrahim et al. [18] studied prospectively the occurrence of VAP and determined the risk factors for VAP and the influence of VAP on patient outcomes. Mortality was higher in patients with VAP than in patients without VAP (45.5% vs. 32.2%, $p < 0.001$), and independent factors associated with mortality were the presence of bacteremia, immunocompromise, higher APACHE II score, and older age.

Patients admitted with a New York Heart Association classification of III or IV are considered to have chronic heart failure. Heart failure has been considered as a high risk for CAP [3] and has been associated with a higher risk for nosocomial pneumonia [19]. In a multicenter study by Cook et al., cardiac disease was found to be an independent risk factor for VAP (risk ratio 2.72, CI 1.05–7.01) [20].

Patients with documented biopsy-proven cirrhosis, documented portal hypertension, episodes of past upper gastrointestinal bleeding attributed to portal hypertension, or previous episodes of hepatic encephalopathy are considered to have chronic hepatopathy. The effect of hepato-pathy on mortality in critically ill patients is thought to be very high. In a prospective study using multiple logistic regression analysis, Osmon et al. identified cirrhosis and the requirement of vasopressors as risk factors for hospital mortality in infected patients requi-ring more than 48 h of intensive care admission [21]. Liebler et al. showed that respiratory complications occurred in 22% of serious upper gastrointestinal bleeding episodes, and more than 50% were pneumonia [22]. Moreover, the mortality rate reached 70% in patients with respiratory complications in contrast to 4% for patients without respiratory complications.

Patients receiving hemodialysis are considered to have chronic renal failure. Advanced age and chronic disease, including chronic renal failure, may diminish physiologic reserve and predispose patients to sepsis [23], and it is known that VAP is the leading infection of ICU acquisition.

2.2
Insult/Infection

Infection is the relationship between the causing microorganism and the host. The severity of this infection can be affected by the site, type, and extent of infection [10]. In the analysis of subgroups of patients from the PROWESS study, Ely et al. showed different mortality rates according to the infection site in the placebo arm [24]. In this study 28-day mortality was 33.6% for lung infection, 30.5% for intra-abdominal infection, 20.9% for urinary tract infection, and 28.5% for infections from another source.

VAP onset is an important issue regarding the associated mortality for ICU patients. Vallés et al., in a prospective cohort study, demonstrated no increased mortality for patients with early-onset VAP. However, patients with late-onset VAP presented an attributable mortality of 25% [25].

Typically, late-onset VAP is caused by high-risk microorganisms [26]. Microorganism virulence is an important key point in the outcome of patients with severe infections such as VAP. Mortality associated with VAP caused by specific microorganisms was evaluated by three matched cohort studies performed by the same group [27–29]. In order to explore mortality caused by microorganism-specific VAP, all episodes needed to be correctly treated, and with a high degree of matching. In patients with VAP by *Acinetobacter baumannii*, the mortality rate was not increased [29]. In contrast, mortality was found to be increased by 22.7% for MRA VAP [28] and 14.2% for *Pseudomonas aeruginosa* VAP [27]. In addition to its susceptibility profile with resistance to several antibiotic classes, a microorganism's virulence factors may contribute to the increased mortality. These virulence factors are of special relevance for *P. aeruginosa* infections [30].

Bacteremia has been related to increased mortality in patients with CAP [31]. Less information is available for bacteremic episodes of VAP. Bacteremic episodes are defined as the presence of the same microorganism in both blood culture and respiratory samples within 48 h in patients with VAP. Bacteremia was related to other sources of infection than the lung. In a cohort study, bacteremia was related to VAP in 17.6% of episodes [32]. After matching for etiology, APACHE II score at admission, diagnostic category, and length of stay before pneumonia, it was found that bacteremia occurred later during the ICU stay, more frequently in previously hospitalized patients, especially those with MRSA, and it was associated with an independent risk for mortality.

2.3
Host Response

The relationship between host, microorganism, and therapy is of special relevance in critically ill patients. Host response has been studied in VAP patients in order to determine the pattern of resolution of clinical variables [33]. After excluding patients with acute respiratory distress syndrome (ARDS), resolution of fever and hypoxemia (defined as a PaO_2/FiO_2 ratio over 250 mmHg) occurred in nearly 75% of patients after 3 days of therapy. VAP resolution is influenced by the causative microorganism being delayed in MRSA VAP episodes regardless of the appropriateness of the initial antibiotic therapy [34].

In a multicenter study, Tejerina et al. determined the risk factors for and outcome of VAP [35]. In patients with VAP, seven complications were found to be related to mortality in a univariate analysis: ARDS, sepsis, shock, acute renal failure, hepatic failure, coagulopathy, and metabolic acidosis. However, only acute renal failure and shock (OR 2.2; 95% CI 1.3–3.8) were associated with mortality in a multivariate analysis. The presence of shock was considered when systolic blood pressure below 90 mmHg was recorded in response to VAP.

In addition to clinical parameters, biomarkers can help physicians to evaluate the response to infection. Seligman et al. studied the value of the kinetics of procalcitonin, C-reactive protein, the clinical pulmonary infection score, and the SOFA score in the outcome of VAP [36]. Biomarkers and scores were evaluated on the of VAP diagnosis and on the fourth day. Survival was directly related to decreasing delta-C-reactive protein and decreasing delta-procalcitonin.

2.4
Organ Dysfunction

Several organs can be affected during a serious infection, which can be presented in variable degrees, from a mild to a severe state. Assessment of organ dysfunction can be made with the SOFA score [37], a tool that evaluates six organs and has been recognized as a valuable prognostic scoring system [38].

Several organs can be affected in the course of a severe infection, and sometimes in parallel [39]. In a multicenter study in ICU patients with CAP, variables independently associated with mortality were shock, high APACHE II score, and the presence of acute renal failure [40]. The lung is the organ most frequently involved in patients with pneumonia. ARDS was diagnosed based on the American–European Consensus Conference Committee criteria [41]. The mortality rate of patients with ARDS seems to be about 44%, and it has not decreased since 1994 when the consensus conference report was published [42]. It is known that VAP can complicate the course of ARDS [43] with an incidence ranging from 37 to 60% [44], but knowledge on this issue is limited when VAP causes ARDS. VAP resolution was found to be delayed in patients with ARDS in the study by Vidaur et al. [33]. In this study, mortality for VAP patients with and without VAP was 35 and 21.3% respectively, without achieving statistical significance. However, the study was weakened by the low number of patients with ARDS (20 ARDS patients).

3
Ventilator-Associated Pneumonia PIRO Score

By mixing the PIRO concept with VAP, a prognostic score system was created [45]. A total of 441 patients with VAP were included in the study. In a univariate analysis, variables found to be associated with mortality in the VAP patients were presence of comorbidities, diagnostic category on admission, age, bacteremia, recent antibiotic therapy, severe hypoxemia, systolic blood pressure below 90 mmHg, and ARDS. A multivariate analysis identified four variables as being independently associated with mortality: presence of comorbidities (predisposition, P), bacteremia (infection insult, I), systolic blood pressure below 90 mmHg or need of vasopressors to maintain blood pressure (response, R), and ARDS (organ dysfunction, O). One point was assigned to each variable, with the VAP PIRO score ranging between 0 and 4.

In the overall population, mortality ranged according to the VAP PIRO score: 9.8% in VAP patients with a VAP PIRO score of 0, 17% for a VAP PIRO score of 1, 52.9% for a VAP PIRO score of 2, 76.5% for a VAP PIRO score of 3, and 93.3% for patients with a VAP PIRO score of 4.

The area under the receiver-operating characteristic (ROC) curve showed high discriminating power (AUROC = 0.81), outperforming the APACHE II score.

The VAP PIRO score was tested in different populations of ICU patients. Some studies have found that VAP in trauma patients is not linked to a high mortality [46, 47]. This statement can be true for the overall population; however, trauma patients with a VAP PIRO score of 4 have a 100% mortality rate (Fig. 1). This figure means that a trauma patient with four points would have VAP with at least one comorbidity, bacteremia due to VAP, a septic shock, and ARDS following VAP. Given this information it seems clear that

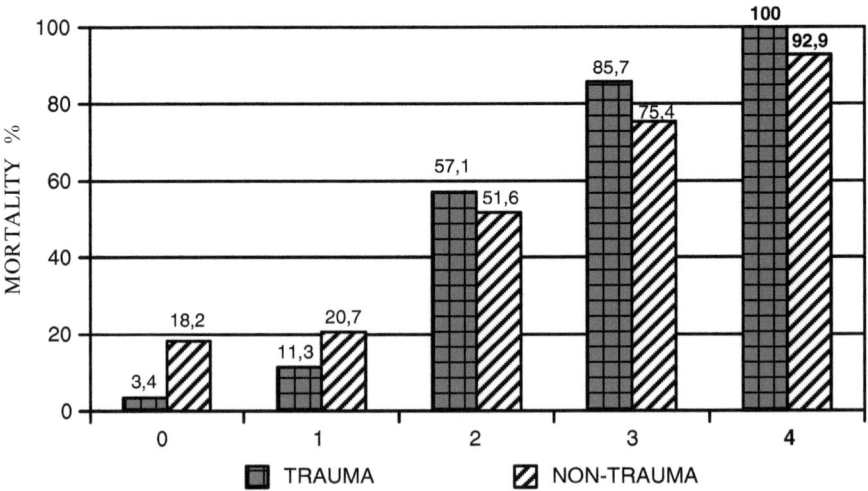

Fig. 1 VAP PIRO score and mortality in patients admitted because of trauma and in nontrauma patients (modified from Lisboa et al. [45])

not all VAP in trauma patients would have similar consequences. The VAP PIRO score showed a similar performance in medical and surgical patients (Fig. 2).

Pneumonia mortality has also been associated with certain etiological agents, especially *P. aeruginosa*, MRSA, and *Acinetobacter baumannii*. These microorganisms are typically found in late-onset VAP. The VAP PIRO score was tested in early-onset and late-onset VAP. Although mortality was higher in late-onset VAP for a given VAP PIRO value, the score showed a good performance in both early-onset and late-onset VAP (Fig. 3).

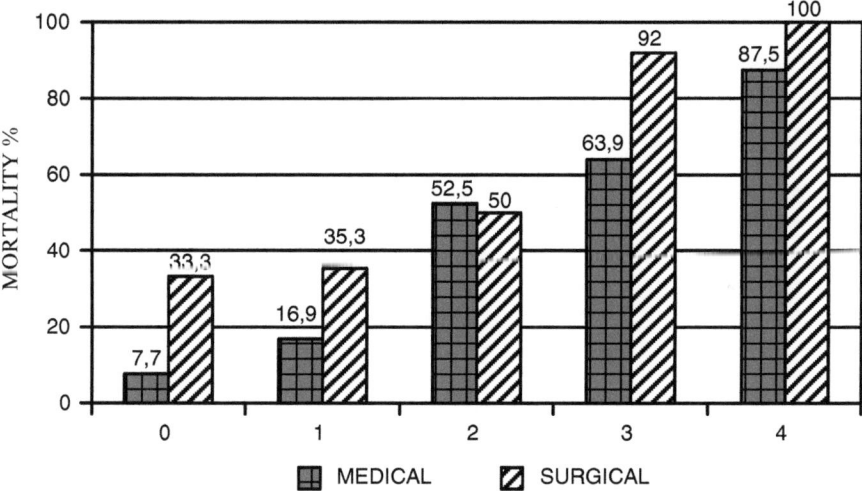

Fig. 2 VAP PIRO score and mortality in patients admitted because of medical and surgical conditions (modified from Lisboa et al. [45])

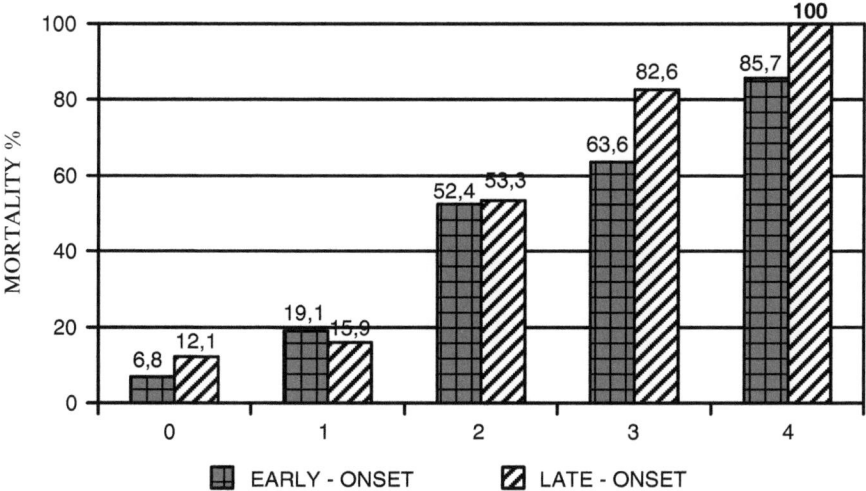

Fig. 3 VAP PIRO score and mortality in patients with early- and late-onset VAP (modified from Lisboa et al. [45])

In a multicenter study in Europe, Koulenti et al. demonstrated that the etiological diagnostics in VAP cases were based mainly on noninvasive techniques [48]. Definite etiology was documented in 75% of patients. The VAP PIRO score stratified both groups of patients, those with and without documented etiology, according to their mortality risk (Fig. 4).

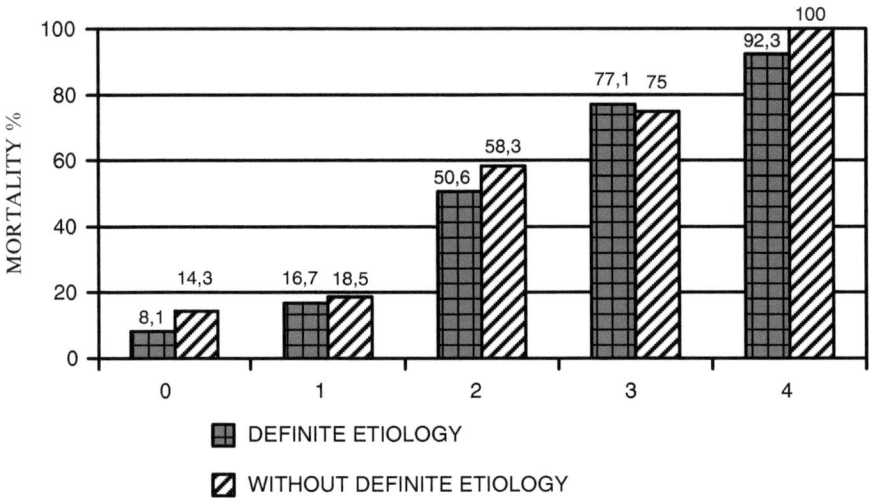

Fig. 4 VAP PIRO score and mortality for patients with or without the presence of a definite etiological agent (modified from Lisboa et al. [45])

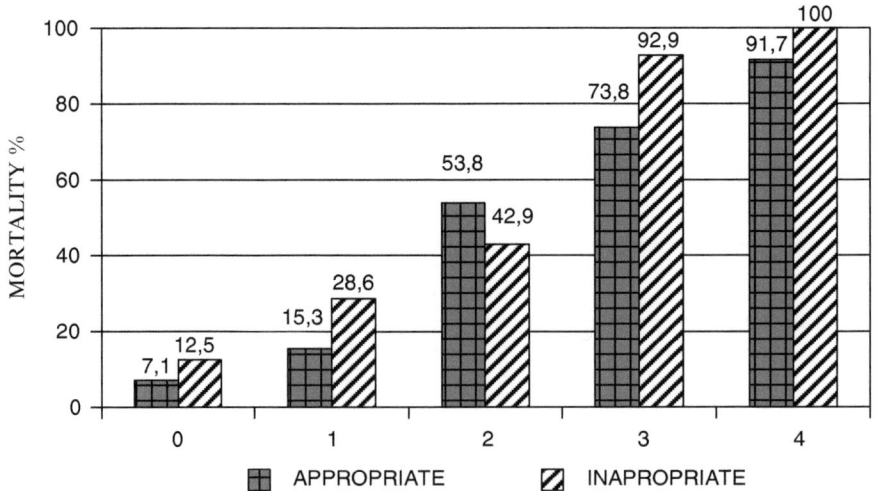

Fig. 5 VAP PIRO score and mortality for patients with or without appropriate empirical antibiotic treatment (modified from Lisboa et al. [45])

Finally, one of the most important factors influencing mortality is the appropriateness of the initial empirical antibiotic therapy. Several studies have found that inappropriate empirical antibiotic treatment is associated with increased mortality [49, 50]. In addition, modification of empirical treatment when microbiological results are available reduces but does not eliminate all associated mortality. Cases with the wrong empirical antibiotic treatment are associated with a higher mortality for a given VAP PIRO score. However, this score stratified correctly the mortality in this subset of patients (Fig. 5).

4
Conclusions

Several scores are available to stratify patients at admission according to their mortality risk; some scores with daily measurements can differentiate whether or not a patient is improving. However, the VAP PIRO score can be useful in daily practice because it allows classification of patients according to their mortality risk with only one measurement on the day of the VAP diagnosis. This simple tool has been tested in different situations and its discriminative power seems to be confirmed.

References

1. Rello J, Diaz E (2003) Pneumonia in the intensive care unit. Crit Care Med 31:2544–2551
2. Chastre J, Fagon JY (2002) Ventilator-associated pneumonia. Am J Respir Crit Care Med 165:867–903
3. Fine MJ, Auble TE, Yealy DM, et al. (1997) A prediction rule to identify low-risk patients with community-acquired pneumonia. N Engl J Med 336:243–250
4. Lim WS, van del Eerden MM, Laing R, et al. (2003) Defining community acquired pneumonia severity on presentation to hospital: an international derivation and validation study. Thorax 58:377–388
5. American Thoracic Society (2005) Guidelines for the management of adults with hospital-acquired, ventilator-associated and healthcare-associated Pneumonia. Am J Respir Crit Care Med 171:388–416
6. http://clinicaltrials.gov/ct2/show/NCT00334828)
7. Rello J, Sole-Violan J, Sa-Borges M, et al. (2005) Pneumonia caused by oxacillin-resistant *Staphylococcus aureus* treated with glycopeptides. Crit Care Med 33:1983–1987
8. Rello J, Rue M, Jubert P, et al. (1997) Survival in patients with nosocomial pneumonia: impact of the severity of illness and the etiologic agent. Crit Care Med 25:1862–1867
9. Bone RC, Balk RA, Cerra FB, et al. (1992) Definitions for sepsis and organ failure and guidelines for the use of innovative therapies in sepsis. The ACCP/SCCM Consensus Conference Committee. American College of Chest Physicians/Society of Critical Care Medicine. Chest 101:1644–1655
10. Levy MM, Fink MP, Marshall JC, et al. (2003) International Sepsis Definitions Conference 2001 SCCM/ESICM/ACCP/ATS/SIS International Sepsis Definitions Conference. Intensive Care Med 29:530–538
11. Moreno RP, Metnitz B, Adler L, et al. (2008) Sepsis mortality prediction based on predisposition, infection and response. Intensive Care Med 34:496–504
12. Shorr AF, Cook D, Jiang X, et al. (2008) Correlates of clinical failure in ventilator-associated pneumonia: insights from a large, randomized trial. J Crit Care 23:64–73

13. Hedrick TL, Smith RL, McElearney ST, et al. (2008) Differences in early- and late-onset ventilator-associated pneumonia between surgical and trauma patients in a combined surgical or trauma intensive care unit. J Trauma 64:714–720
14. Myny D, Depuydt P, Colardyn F, Blot S (2005) Ventilator-associated pneumonia in a tertiary care ICU: analysis of risk factors for acquisition and mortality. Acta Clin Belg 60:114–121
15. National Heart, Lung, and Blood Institute. Morbidity & mortality: chartbook on cardiovascular, lung, and blood diseases. Bethesda, MD: US Department of Health and Human Services, Public Health Service, National Institutes of Health; 1998. Available from: URL: http://www.nhlbi.nih.gov/nhlbi/seiin//other/cht-book/htm
16. Rabe K, Hurd S, Anzueto A, et al. (2007) Global strategy for the diagnosis, management, and prevention of chronic obstructive pulmonary disease (GOLD). Am J Respir Crit Care Med 176:532–555
17. Nseir S, Di Pompeo C, Soubrier S, et al. (2005) Impact of ventilator-associated pneumonia on outcome in patients with COPD. Chest 128:1650–1656
18. Ibrahim EH, Tracy L, Hill C, et al. (2001) The occurrence of ventilator-associated pneumonia in a community hospital. Risk factors and clinical outcomes. Chest 120:555–561
19. Mistiaen W, Visseres D (2008) The risk of postoperative pulmonary or pleural complications after aortic valve replacement is low in elderly patients: an observational study. Aust J Physiother 54:119–124
20. Cook DJ, Walter SD, Cook RJ, et al. (1998) Incidence of and risk factors for ventilator-associated pneumonia in critically ill patients. Ann Int Med 129:433–440
21. Osmon S, Warren D, Seiler SM, et al. (2003) The influence of infection on hospital mortality for patients requiring >48 h of intensive care. Chest 124:1021–1029
22. Liebler JM, Benner K, Putnam T, Vollmer WM (1991) Respiratory complications in critically ill medical patients with acute upper gastrointestinal bleeding. Crit Care Med 19:1152–1157
23. Tran DD, Groeneveld AB, van der Meulen J, et al. (1990) Age, chronic disease, sepsis, organ system failure, and mortality in a medical intensive care unit. Crit Care Med 18:474–479
24. Ely EW, Laterre PF, Angus DC, et al. (2003) Drotrecogin alfa (activated) administration across clinically important subgroups of patients with severe sepsis. Crit Care Med 31:12–19
25. Vallés J, Pobo A, García-Esquirol O, et al. (2007) Excess ICU mortality attributable to ventilator-associated pneumonia: the role of early vs late onset. Intensive Care Med 33:1363–1368
26. Diaz E, Muñoz E, Agbaht, K, Rello J (2007) Management of ventilator-associated pneumonia caused by multiresistant bactéria. Curr Opin Crit Care 13:45–50
27. Rello J, Jubert P, Vallés J, et al. (1996) Evaluation of outcome for intubated patients with pneumonia due to *Pseudomonas aeruginosa*. Clin Infect Dis 23:973–978
28. Rello J, Sole-Violan J, Sa-Borges M, et al. (2005) Pneumonia caused by oxacillin-resistant *Staphylococcus aureus* treated with glycopeptides. Crit Care Med 33:1983–1987
29. Garnacho J, Sole-Violan J, Sa-Borges M, et al. (2003) Clinical impact of pneumonia caused by *Acinetobacter baumannii* in intubated patients: a matched cohort study. Crit Care Med 31:2478–2482
30. Schulert GS, Feltman H, Rabin SD, et al. (2003) Secretion of the toxin ExoU is a marker for highly virulent *Pseudomonas aeruginosa* isolates obtained from patients with hospital-acquired pneumonia. J Infect Dis 188:1695–706
31. Garcia-Vidal C, Fernández-Sabé N, Carratalà J, et al. (2008) Early mortality in patients with community-acquired pneumonia: causes and risk factors. Eur Respir J 32:733–739
32. Agbath K, Diaz E, Muñoz E, et al. (2007) Bacteremia in patients with ventilator-associated pneumonia is associated with increased mortality: A study comparing bacteremic vs. nonbacteremic ventilator-associated pneumonia. Crit Care Med 35:2215–2226
33. Vidaur L, Gualis B, Rodriguez A, et al. (2005) Clinical resolution in patients with suspicion of ventilator-associated pneumonia: A cohort study comparing patients with and without acute respiratory distress syndrome. Crit Care Med 33:1248–1253

34. Vidaur L, Planas K, Sierra R, et al. (2008) Ventilator-associated pneumonia: impacto f organisms on clinical resolution and medical resources utilization. Chest 133:625–632
35. Tejerina E, Frutos-Vivar F, Restrepo MI, et al. (2006) Incidence, risk factors, and outcome of ventilator-associated pneumonia. J Crit Care 21:56–65
36. Seligman R, Meisner M, Lisboa TC, et al. (2006) Decreases in procalcitonin and C-reactive protein are strong predictors of survival in ventilator-associated pneumonia. Crit Care 10:R125
37. Vincent JL, de Mendonça A, Cantraine F, et al. (1998) Use of the SOFA score to assess the incidence of organ dysfunction failure in intensive care units: Results of a multicentric prospective study. Crit Care Med 26:1793–180
38. Lopes Ferreira F, Peres Bota D, Bross A, et al. (2001) Serial evaluation of the SOFA score to predict outcome JAMA 286:1754–1758
39. Steinvall I, Bak Z, Sjoberg F (2008) Acute kidney inury is common, parallels organ dysfunction or failure, and carries appreciable mortality in patients with major burns: a prospective exploratory cohort study. Crit Care 12(5):R124
40. Rodriguez A, Lisboa T, Blot S, et al. (2009) Mortality in ICU patients with bacterial community-acquired pneumonia: when antibiotics are not enough. Intensive Care Med 35:430–438
41. Bernard GR, Artigas A, Brigham KL et al. (1994) The American–European Consensus Conference on ARDS. Definitions, mechanisms, relevant outcomes, and clinical trial coordination. Am J Respir Crit Care Med 149: 818–824
42. Phua J, Badia JR, Adhikari NK, et al. (2009) Has mortality from acute respiratory distress syndrome decreased over time? A systematic review. Am J Respir Crit Care Med 179(3): 220–227
43. Markowicz P, Wolff M, Djedaïni K, et al. (2000) Multicenter prospective study of ventilator-associated pneumonia during acute respiratory distress syndrome. Incidence, prognosis, and risk factors. ARDS Study Group. Am J Respir Crit Care Med 161:1942–1948
44. Wunderink RG, Waterer GW (2002) Pneumonia complicating the acute respiratory distress syndrome. Sem Respir Crit Care Med 23:443–448
45. Lisboa T, Diaz E, Sa-Borges M, et al. (2008) The ventilator-associated pneumonia PIRO score: a tool for predicting ICU mortality and helath-care resources use in ventilator-associated pneumonia. Chest 134:1208–1216
46. Baker AM, Meredith JW, Haponik EF (1996) Pneumonia in intubated trauma patients. Microbiology and outcomes. Am J Respir Crit Care Med 153:343–349
47. Hedrick T, Smith R, McElearney S, et al. (2008) Difference in early- and late-onset ventilator-associated pneumonia between surgical and trauma patients in a combined surgical or trauma intensive care unit. J Trauma 64:714–720
48. Koulenti D, Lisboa T, Brun-Buisson C, et al. (2009) The Spectrum of Practice in the Diagnosis of Nosocomial Pneumonia in Patients Requiring Mechanical Ventilation in European ICUs. Crit Care Med (in press)
49. Rello J, Gallego M, Mariscal D, et al. (1997) The value of routine microbial investigation in ventilator-associated pneumonia. Am J Respir Crit Care Med 156:196–200
50. Teixeira PJ, Seligman R, Hertz FT, et al. (2007) Inadequate treatment of ventilator-associated pneumonia: risk factors and impact on outcomes. J Hosp Infect 65:361–367

A PIRO-Based Approach for Severity Assessment in Community-Acquired Pneumonia

Thiago Lisboa, Alejandro Rodríguez, and Jordi Rello

1 Introduction

Community-acquired pneumonia (CAP) is an acute illness with clinical features of a lower respiratory tract infection characterized by new radiological shadowing and no other explanation for the illness. There are many definitions of severe CAP, and the best way to define severity is controversial. Pragmatically, severe CAP can be defined as a disease that necessitates admission to an intensive care unit (ICU) [1, 2], which is the definition used in many clinical trials. However, more systematic criteria that permit integration of objective measurements into the assessment and avoid variation caused by differing ICU admittance policies across institutions are desirable [3, 4].

Approximately four million adults develop CAP annually in the United States [5]. Among hospitalized CAP patients in Europe and the United States, the rates of severe CAP range from 6.6 to 16.7% [6–10]. Mortality from severe CAP is high worldwide, with pneumonia/influenza as the eighth leading cause of death in the United States, accounting for 0.3% of deaths in 2004 [5]. Severe CAP mortality ranges from 20 to 50%, depending on the definition criteria [11, 12].

Severe CAP is a progressive disease, and in the event of evolution from a local to a systemic infection, the following spectrum of sepsis-related complications may develop (Fig. 1): sepsis, severe sepsis, septic shock, and multiple organ dysfunction. Approximately 50% of CAP admissions to Spanish ICUs are associated with septic shock [13]. Progression of severe CAP is associated with hypercoagulation, hypotension, alteration of the microcirculation, and ultimately multiple organ dysfunction. Nearly all patients who die as a consequence of severe CAP develop severe sepsis, septic shock, or organ dysfunction during the disease evolution.

T. Lisboa (✉)
Critical Care Department, Joan XXIII University Hospital, University Rovira i Virgili,
Institut Pere Virgili, CIBER Enfermedades Respiratorias (CIBERes),
Carrer Dr. Mallafre Guasch 4 (43007), Tarragona, Spain
e-mail: tlisboa@hotmail.com

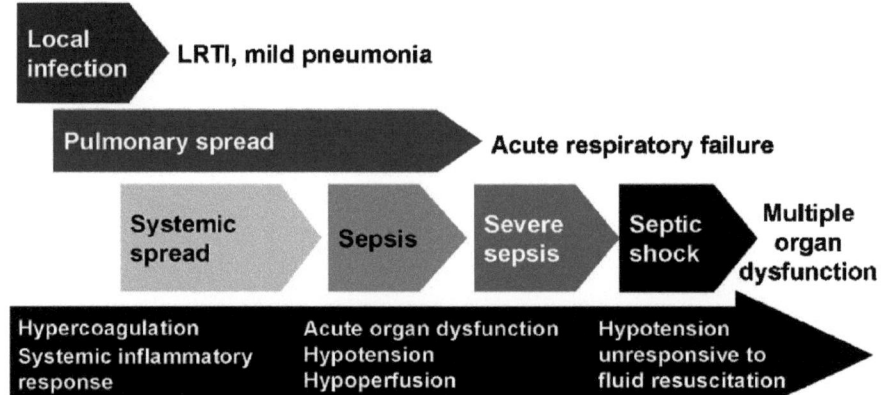

Fig. 1 Community-acquired pneumonia as a systemic and progressive disease

2
Assessing Severity in CAP Patients: Why and How Is PIRO Useful?

Early identification of patients at risk of severe CAP can aid patient management. Although age is an important risk factor for the development of CAP, comorbidities also play an important part in determining the risk for pneumonia and disease severity. Physicians should therefore take into account any history of chronic obstructive pulmonary disease (COPD), renal insufficiency/dialysis, chronic heart failure, coronary artery disease, diabetes mellitus, malignancy, chronic neurologic disease, and chronic liver disease/alcohol abuse when they determine patient management. In patients older than 60 years, risk is further increased by the presence of asthma, alcoholism, or immunosuppression, and it is also increased in institutionalized patients [14].

Other factors that have been implicated in increasing mortality in severe CAP patients include male sex and the development of acute respiratory failure, severe sepsis/septic shock, and bacteremia [15]. Some specific pathogens also carry an increased risk of severe CAP. The most prevalent pathogen associated with severe CAP, namely, *Streptococcus pneumoniae*, is responsible for two-thirds of CAP-related deaths. Signs of disease progression during the first 72 h after hospital admission are also associated with an increased risk of death. A rapid radiological progression of pulmonary infiltrates predicts a poor outcome and is associated with shock and higher mortality [16]. For patients without comorbidities, the presence of multilobar consolidation and the need for mechanical ventilation or inotropic support are associated with greater disease severity and higher mortality rates [17].

However, despite of clinical importance, to date no score has appropriately assessed severity and stratified risk in ICU patients with a diagnosis of severe CAP. Scores are mainly designed to be used in the emergency room setting and to allow a prompt hospital discharge, neglecting the subpopulation at higher risk of mortality.

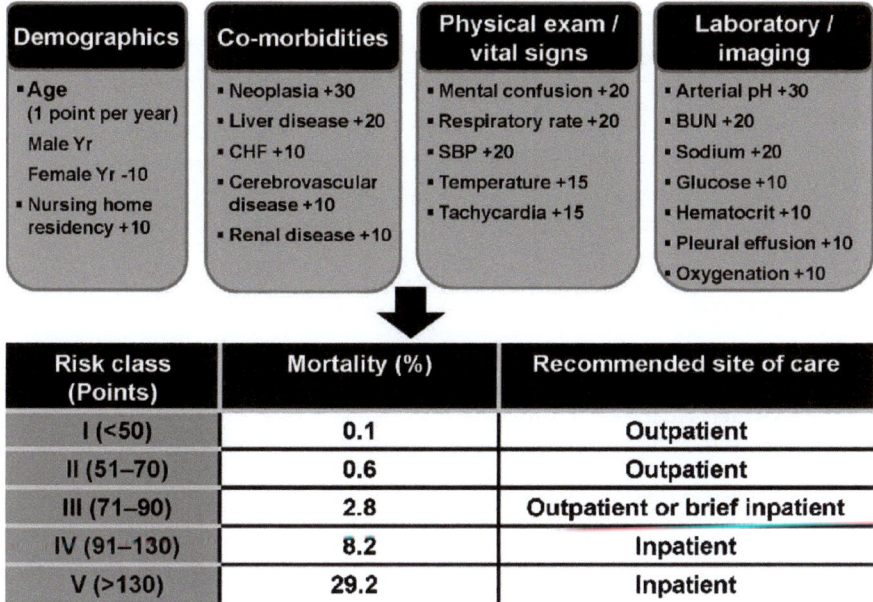

Fig. 2 Pneumonia Severity Index (PSI) Score and Interpretation

There are various severity assessment tools available, including the Pneumonia Severity Index (PSI) [18] and the British Thoracic Society CURB-65 (confusion, urea, respiratory rate, blood pressure, age ≥65 years) score [19]. The PSI was developed primarily to identify patients who can safely be treated as outpatients (Fig. 2). According to this score, the main determinants of pneumonia severity are increasing age, comorbidity, and vital sign abnormalities. The calculation of the PSI score also requires laboratory, blood gas, and chest radiography data, making this a more problematic set of tests to perform in the emergency room setting.

The PSI has been convincingly validated in several studies, and it allows the confident separation of patients with a mortality risk of up to 3% (PSI classes I–III) from those with risks of 8% (PSI class IV) and 35% (PSI class V). However, it should be noted that although the PSI takes into account renal, cardiac, cardiovascular, or hepatic disease and malignancy, it does not include COPD or diabetes as risk factors. The PSI is therefore a useful tool for identifying patients who can be discharged safely and can receive home treatment with antibiotics. The PSI has also been useful in demonstrating equivalence between different empirical antibiotics, and in showing that delaying appropriate antibiotics worsens survival in patients with classes IV–V pneumococcal bacteremic pneumonia [20]. However, PSI underestimates mortality risk in younger patients and its use in the ICU has not been adequately validated.

In contrast to the complexity of the PSI, the British Thoracic Society CURB-65 system uses simple clinical measures and a single laboratory investigation (blood urea), which is readily available in most hospitals (Table 1) [19]. These scores are useful in determining which patients may be treated at home safely, and they can flag certain hospitalized patients

Table 1 British Thoracic Society CURB-65 criteria

*C*onfusion	1 point
*U*rea (>7 mmol/ L^{-1})	1 point
*R*espiratory rate (≥30 min^{-1})	1 point
*B*lood pressure (SBP < 90 mmHg or DBP ≤ 60 mmHg)	1 point
Age (≥65 years)	1 point
0–1: Outpatient management	
2: Short hospital stay/supervised outpatient	
3–5: Hospital management, assess for ICU	

Table 2 Infectious Diseases Society of America/American Thoracic Society criteria

Major criteria
Invasive mechanical ventilation
Septic shock with the need for vasopressors
Minor criteria (at least three of these)
Respiratory rate ≥30 breaths/min
PaO_2/FiO_2 ratio ≤ 250
Multilobar infiltrates
New onset confusion/disorientation
Uremia (BUN level ≥20 mg dL^{-1})
Leukopenia (WBC count < 4,000 cells mm^3)
Thrombocytopenia (platelets < 100,000 cells mm^3)
Hypothermia (core temperature < 36 °C)
Hypotension requiring aggressive fluid resuscitation

BUN blood urea nitrogen; *WBC* white blood cell

for careful scrutiny and for admission to the ICU if their condition deteriorates. However, these tools have limitations in identifying all patients with severe pneumonia who require ICU admission.

The Infectious Diseases Society of America (IDSA)/American Thoracic Society (ATS) recently reviewed risk factors and developed objective major and minor criteria to identify patients who require direct admission to an ICU [1]. The most up-to-date definitions use the following as absolute indicators for direct admission to an ICU: need for invasive mechanical ventilation, septic shock, or requiring vasopressors (Table 2). Validation of the use of these objective criteria in a large population of patients indicated that CURB-65 can be used as an alternative to PSI to identify low-risk patients, and confirmed the ability of the IDSA/ATS guidelines to predict disease severity [9].

Recently, Charles et al. [21] developed a tool for predicting which CAP patients would require intensive respiratory support or vasopressors. The SMART-COP system utilizes the following variables: *s*ystolic blood pressure, *m*ultilobar opacities, low *a*lbumin levels, *r*espiratory rate (age adjusted), *t*achycardia, *c*onfusion, low *o*xygen (age adjusted), and arterial *p*H (pH < 7.35). SMART-COP may be a useful alternative for severity assessment in the emergency setting, identifying patients more likely to need intensive respiratory support and vasopressors.

Although factors reflecting acute respiratory failure and severe sepsis or septic shock are independent predictors of severity in CAP [15], and sepsis severity at admission significantly affects outcome [22], such factors have not been systematically implemented into risk classification systems for CAP patients.

In 2003, a consensus conference provided the basis for introducing the PIRO concept as a hypothesis-generating model for future research [23]. According to this concept, septic patients are classified according to four domains: predisposition (chronic illness, age and comorbidities); insult (injury, bacteremia, endotoxin); response (neutropenia, hypoxemia, shock), and organ dysfunction.

The complexity of pneumonia might be better understood after assessment of these aspects of the disease. Predisposition factors such as the genetic profile of an individual are likely to be a major determinant of the lifetime predisposition to sepsis, and progress continues to be made in identifying relevant candidate genes. However, the presence of comorbid conditions and age are also important predisposing factors that affect outcomes in pneumonia. The site of infection and the nature and spread of the pathogen within the body are also important features, including the presence of bacteremia and the pattern of radiological spread. Although some elements of the variables that affect the host response to infection are easy to identify (age, nutritional status, sex, comorbid conditions etc.), others are more complex and arise from interactions between inflammation, coagulation, and sepsis. Development of shock and hypoxemia are important factors related to the host response to infection. Use of biomarkers might help in identifying response patterns, thereby helping to assess severity. Finally, development of organ dysfunction is a clear sign of poor evolution [4].

In an attempt to address the need to identify ICU CAP patients at high risk, using readily available clinical data, a new form of classification has been proposed based on the PIRO system.

3
The CAP PIRO Score

We have developed a PIRO concept-based score (CAP PIRO score) [24] that is applicable in the setting of severe CAP. To construct this score we considered a database from 33 Spanish ICUs (CAPUCI database) [23] including consecutive patients aged 18 years or older with conclusive evidence of pneumonia as the primary diagnosis, as confirmed by chest radiographs and clinical findings. The study focused on patients admitted to the ICU and excluded patients with respiratory infection other than pneumonia (e.g., exacerbation of COPD), long-term care facility and nursing-home-associated pneumonia, or recent (<3 months) hospitalization.

The variables used in the new score (age; COPD; immunocompromise; multilobar opacities on chest X-ray; shock; severe hypoxemia and acute renal failure) were selected

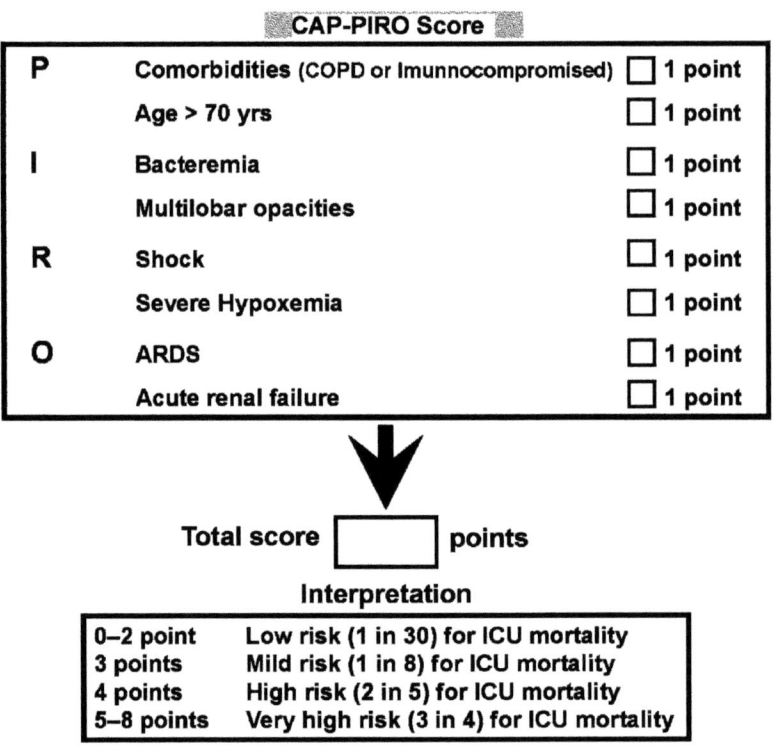

Fig. 3 The CAP PIRO Score for severity assessment in SCAP

from the current literature as being more significant in CAP prognosis or because they were considered to have clinical importance (bacteremia and acute respiratory distress syndrome [ARDS]). A new clinical severity assessment score (PIRO score for CAP) is calculated based on these variables, determined within 24 h after ICU admission (Fig. 3).

4
Selection of Variables

4.1
Predisposition

Current opinion holds that the genetic makeup of an individual is likely to be a major determinant of their lifetime predisposition to sepsis, and progress continues to be made in identifying relevant candidate genes [15, 25]. The role of genetic predisposition and the clinical implications of specific genetic variations are still unclear. However, predisposing factors such as age, immunocompromise, or comorbidities are associated with an increased risk of severe CAP. The CAP PIRO Score identified age (odds ratio [OR] = 1.9,

95% confidence interval [CI] = 1.3–2.9) and the presence of comorbidities (COPD and immunocompromise) (OR = 1.9, 95% CI = 1.3–2.8) as predisposing factors affecting outcome in severe CAP patients admitted to the ICU [24].

Emerging evidence suggests that critically ill patients with severe CAP and COPD are more likely to need mechanical ventilation and carry an increased risk of mortality [26, 27]. COPD proved to be an important risk factor for mortality. In COPD patients, both mechanical ventilation (OR = 2.78, 95% CI = 1.63–4.74) and ICU mortality (OR = 1.58, 95% CI = 1.01–1.43) rates were higher than in non-COPD patients [27]. The ICU mortality rate was 39% in COPD patients initially intubated, and 50% in those who did not respond to noninvasive ventilation.

Patients with a history of COPD are likely to have more severe signs at presentation: septic shock; tachypnea; lower pH, partial oxygen tension, and oxygen saturation; and greater partial carbon dioxide tension. COPD is more common in patients with increasing age, in male patients, and in patients with diabetes or chronic heart failure [26].

The relationships between immunocompromise and risk for infectious diseases are well described. The impact of immunocompromise on outcomes of severe CAP is suggested by CAP PIRO Score. Immunoglobulin deficiency is known to predispose patients to pneumonia, but CAP can be prevented by administration of immunoglobulins. Immunization against *S. pneumoniae* is also a valid strategy for prevention. Unfortunately, other immunocompromise situations do not allow effective prevention measures, and it is important to have early identification of these patients as well as early recognition of the higher risk for worse outcomes in order to assure a prompt and appropriate management of severe CAP.

The impact of age on CAP outcomes has been described. Numerous factors can contribute to higher mortality in older patients, such as difficulties in diagnosis and delay in starting appropriate treatment. Moreover, older patients also present with a higher frequency of comorbid illnesses and immune function alterations secondary to advanced age and comorbidities [28]. Kothe et al. described different risk factors for mortality in young and old patients, with age being associated with a higher risk of mortality in those older than 65 years [29].

4.2
Insult

The site of infection and the nature and spread of the pathogen within the body are also important features. The CAP PIRO score identified the presence of bacteremia (OR = 1.8, 95% CI = 1.1–2.8) and the presence of multilobar compromise on chest X-rays (OR = 4.2, 95% CI = 2.7–6.3) – variables included in the "insult" category of the PIRO concept – as being associated with worse outcomes in severe CAP patients [24].

The importance of detecting bacteremic episodes may be underestimated in most studies because of the low sensitivity of conventional blood culture methods. Improvements in bacteremia detection may allow for a more precise evaluation of the true effect of systemic invasion on outcomes in severe CAP. Recent data suggest that this is true for *S. pneumoniae* severe CAP episodes. A preliminary study demonstrated the feasibility of a noncommercial quantitative real-time polymerase chain reaction to identify *S. pneumoniae* DNA in whole blood [30]. A subsequent prospective study [31] demonstrated that this technique was able to identify "hidden" bloodstream invasion in patients with pneumococcal pneumonia. Moreover, a "high" bacterial burden (> 1,000 copies mL^{-1}) at the time of emergency department presentation was highly correlated with subsequent septic shock, need for Intensive respiratory or vasopressors support (IRVS), and 28-day mortality [31]. Whereas previous studies have suggested that severe sepsis is related to delay in therapy or an exaggerated host inflammatory response, this study suggests for the first time that insult, the bacterial burden, plays a key role in the development of severe sepsis and multiorgan system failure.

In addition to the effect of local bacterial proliferation, the emergence of a community-acquired methicillin-resistant *Staphylococcus aureus* (MRSA) strain in the United States has restimulated concern about the role of exotoxins and other bacterial products in the pathogenesis of severe CAP, such as Panton-Valentine leukocidin and hematoxin, and they may be useful in cavitary pneumonias which are more likely to be caused by community-acquired MRSA. The role of toxins such as pneumolysin in the pathophysiology of pneumococcal pneumonia, and new therapeutic possibilities targeting these toxins should also be further assessed.

The presence of multilobar opacities on chest X-rays was also associated with severity in severe CAP, and it is included in the CAP PIRO score. Feldman et al. found that the presence of multilobar opacities is an independent risk factor for mortality in CAP patients [32]. Moreover, an association between the worsening of radiological infiltrates and the development of septic shock and mortality was recently described [16, 33], emphasizing the importance of radiological findings as prognostic factors in severe CAP.

4.3
Response

Some elements of the variables that affect the host response to infection are complex and arise from interactions between inflammation, coagulation, and sepsis. Hypoxemia is one of the cardinal signs of severe CAP. In conjunction, the presence of hypotension and shock are important points when assessing severity in severe CAP patients. Severe hypoxemia (OR = 19.9, 95% CI = 8.6–46.1) and shock (OR = 12.4, 95% CI = 7.3–21.2) were identified as independent factors associated with worse outcomes in the CAP PIRO score [24].

Beyond the expected prognosis suggested by the relationship between the presence of hypoxemia and shock — necessitating intensive respiratory and hemodynamic support — and worse outcomes in severe CAP, identification of these patients might have therapeutic implications. Interestingly, administration of macrolides [34] has been associated with improved survival in patients with a systolic blood pressure under 90 mmHg. This effect is independent of the antimicrobial activity of macrolides, and seems to be associated with the immunomodulatory effects on the cytokine response to macrolides [35]. This effect is the likely explanation for the improved survival found with macrolide combination therapy of bacteremic pneumococcal pneumonia.

Late deaths are associated with persistent respiratory failure. Interestingly, a meta-analysis of patients with CAP [35] suggested that adding steroids to the treatment of patients with severe CAP was associated with a significantly reduced risk of respiratory failure. Although steroids are recommended (2C) by the Sepsis Surviving Campaign [36] for patients with refractory shock, the benefit specifically in severe CAP patients could be more than simply improving hemodynamics. Further studies should clarify what patients are more likely to benefit from steroids and how does it affect long–term outcomes [37].

Biomarkers such as cytokines, C-reactive protein, and procalcitonin, identified as markers of host response to sepsis, may improve traditional scoring factors in predicting outcomes, but this approach has yet to be validated.

4.4
Organ Failure

We found two organ dysfunctions related with outcomes in severe CAP patients: ARDS (OR = 70.1) and acute renal failure (OR = 12.6) were included in the CAP PIRO score [24]. Death within 72 h of ICU admission is typically associated with shock and respiratory failure and later mortality is typically associated with development of organ failure. When organ failure is present at admission or develops within 24 h from ICU admission, the prognosis is even worse. Recently, it was described that presence of acute renal failure is independently associated with higher mortality (HR = 3.4) in patients with an appropriate antibiotic treatment [38]. The presence of ARDS early in the course of pneumonia may be associated with either a severe compromise of pulmonary function or with an exaggerated systemic inflammatory response. However, independently of the responsible mechanism, development of ARDS affects negatively the prognosis of severe CAP patients [23, 39].

The incorporation of the SOFA score, newer functional biomarkers (e.g., cortisol), and other organ dysfunctions (e.g., coagulation, hepatic) in severe CAP prognosis systems should be further evaluated.

5
How Does This Score Perform?

The CAP PIRO score was significantly associated with mortality in severe CAP patients. A cross-validation model revealed an excellent correlation between increasing CAP PIRO score and mortality rate ($p < 0.001$) with a good calibration. Moreover, the model presented a good discrimination ability (area under ROC curve = 0.88, 95% CI = 0.83–0.90) and outperformed the APACHE II score at admission ($p < 0.05$) and the ATS major criteria ($p < 0.05$) for mortality prediction. A CAP PIRO score of 4 points or more was associated with the best performance in predicting 28-day mortality with a sensitivity of 86% and specificity of 76%.

Analysis of the points obtained in the CAP PIRO score allowed identification of four levels of risk for mortality: (a) low, 0–2 points; (b) mild, 3 points; (c) high, 4 points; and (d) very high, 5–8 points (Fig. 4). Moreover, the CAP PIRO score was also associated with

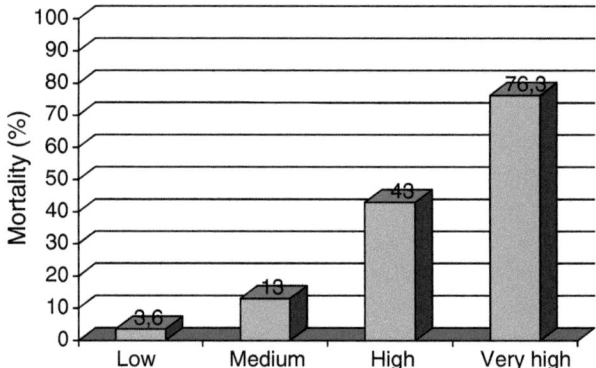

Fig. 4 Mortality according to severity level assessed by CAP PIRO Score

increased healthcare resource utilization in CAP patients admitted to an ICU, considering the duration of mechanical ventilation and length of stay ($p < 0.001$).

Furthermore, the predictive ability of the CAP PIRO score was not affected by etiology. A subanalysis of only pneumococcal pneumonia demonstrated that the score retains a good discriminative and predictive ability. Another subanalysis excluded immunocompromised patients and found similar results.

6
What Next? The Future of the CAP PIRO Score

The CAP PIRO score is the first score specifically designed for severity assessment in severe CAP in an ICU setting. It is a simple tool with an excellent performance in predicting outcomes in severe CAP patients admitted to the ICU. The variables included are easily available. Patients are easily risk stratified into different levels of severity, taking into account progressive rates of mortality and medical resource utilization in the ICU. It includes aspects neglected in the available severity assessment tools, as it is designed for a specific group of patients.

Optimization of therapy based on this classification is a strategy that should be evaluated (see Chapter "CAP Management based on the PIRO System: A new therapeutic paradigm"), since higher-risk patients may benefit from more aggressive strategies or adjuvant therapy. As it appropriately stratifies patients in such different risk groups, clinical trials designed to evaluate therapeutic strategies for severe CAP patients should use this tool in an analysis of outcomes. It should probably replace the misused APACHE II score in defining subgroups who could benefit more from specific adjuvant therapies. It may also help to stratify patients with a PSI above 130 (class V) into different categories of severity.

The CAP PIRO score may be useful for pharmacoeconomic or outcome comparisons, and for selecting candidates for adjunctive therapy in future clinical trials.

References

1. Mandell LA, Wunderink RG, Anzueto A, Bartlett JG, Campbell GD, Dean NC, Dowell SF, File TM Jr, Musher DM, Niederman MS, Torres A, Whitney CG. Infectious Diseases Society of America; American Thoracic Society: Infectious Diseases Society of America/American Thoracic Society consensus guidelines on the management of community-acquired pneumonia in adults. *Clin Infect Dis* 2007; 44(Suppl 2):S27–S72
2. Kamath AV, Myint PK. Recognising and managing severe community acquired pneumonia. *Br J Hosp Med* 2006; 26:76–78
3. Oosterheert JJ, Bonten MJ, Hak E, Schneider MM, Hoepelman AI. Severe community-acquired pneumonia: what's in a name? *Curr Opin Infect Dis* 2003; 16:153–159
4. Rello J: Demographics, guidelines and clinical experience in severe community-acquired pneumonia. *Crit Care* 2008; 12(Suppl 6):S2
5. Aliberti S, Amir A, Peyrani P, et al.: Incidence, etiology timing and risk factors for clinical failure in hospitalized patients with community-acquired pneumonia. *Chest* 2008; 134:955–962
6. Marrie TJ, Shariatzadeh MR. Community-acquired pneumonia requiring admission to an intensive care unit: a descriptive study. *Medicine* (Baltimore) 2007; 86:103–111
7. Bauer TT, Welte T, Ernen C, Schlosser BM, Thate-Waschke I, de Zeeuw J, Schultze-Werninghaus G. Cost analyses of community-acquired pneumonia from the hospital perspective. *Chest* 2005; 128:2238–2246
8. España PP, Capelastegui A, Gorordo I, Esteban C, Oribe M, Ortega M, Bilbao A, Quintana JM. Development and validation of a clinical prediction rule for severe community-acquired pneumonia. *Am J Respir Crit Care Med* 2006; 174:1249–1256
9. Ewig S, de Roux A, Bauer T, García E, Mensa J, Niederman M, Torres A. Validation of predictive rules and indices of severity for community acquired pneumonia. *Thorax* 2004; 59:421–4277
10. Riley PD, Aronsky D, Dean NC. Validation of the 2001 American Thoracic Society criteria for severe community-acquired pneumonia. *Crit Care Med* 2004; 32:2398–2402
11. Woodhead MA, Macfarlane JT, Rodgers FG, Laverick A, Pilkington R, Macrae AD. Aetiology and outcome of severe community-acquired pneumonia. *J Infect* 1985; 10:204–210
12. Moine P, Vercken JB, Chevret S, Chastang C, Gajdos P. Severe community-acquired pneumonia. Etiology, epidemiology, and prognosis factors. French Study Group for community-acquired pneumonia in the intensive care unit. *Chest* 1994; 105:1487–1495
13. Rodríguez A, Mendia A, Sirvent JM, Barcenilla F, de la Torre-Prados MV, Solé-Violán J, Rello J. CAPUCI Study Group: Combination antibiotic therapy improves survival in patients with community-acquired pneumonia and shock. *Crit Care Med* 2007; 35:1493–1498
14. Mandell LA. Epidemiology and etiology of community-acquired pneumonia. *Infect Dis Clin N Am* 2004; 18:761–776
15. Neuhaus T, Ewig S, Defining severe community-acquired pneumonia. *Med Clin N Am* 2001; 85:1413–1425
16. Lisboa T, Blot S, Waterer GW, Canalis E, de Mendoza D, Rodriguez A, Rello J. Community-acquired pneumonia intensive care units (CAPUCI) study investigators: radiological progression of pulmonary infiltrates predicts a worse prognosis in severe community-acquired pneumonia than bacteremia. *Chest* 2009; 135:165–172
17. Feldman C, Viljoen E, Morar R, Richards G, Sawyer L, Goolam Mahomed A. Prognostic factors in severe community-acquired pneumonia in patients without co-morbid illness. *Respirology* 2001; 6:323–330

18. Fine MJ, Auble TE, Yealy DM, Hanusa BH, Weissfeld LA, Singer DE, Coley CM, Marrie TJ, Kapoor WN. A prediction rule to identify low-risk patients with community-acquired pneumonia. *N Engl J Med* 1997; 336:243–250
19. Lim WS, van der Eerden MM, Laing R, Boersma WG, Karalus N, Town GI, Lewis SA, Macfarlane JT. Defining community acquired pneumonia severity on presentation to hospital: an international derivation and validation study. *Thorax* 2003; 58:377–382
20. Spindler C, Ortqvist A. Prognostic score systems and community-acquired bacteraemic pneumococcal pneumonia. *Eur Respir J* 2006; 28:816–823
21. Charles PG, Wolfe R, Whitby M, Fine MJ, Fuller AJ, Stirling R, Wright AA, Ramirez JA, Christiansen KJ, Waterer GW, Pierce RJ, Armstrong JG, Korman TM, Holmes P, Obrosky DS, Peyrani P, Johnson B, Hooy M. Australian Community-Acquired Pneumonia Study Collaboration, Grayson ML: SMART-COP: a tool for predicting the need for intensive respiratory or vasopressor support in community-acquired pneumonia. *Clin Infect Dis* 2008; 47:375–384
22. Schaaf B, Kruse J, Rupp J, Reinert RR, Droemann D, Zabel P, Ewig S, Dalhoff K. Sepsis severity predicts outcome in community-acquired pneumococcal pneumonia. *Eur Respir J* 2007; 30:517–524
23. Levy MM, Fink MP, Marshall JC, et al. 2001 SCCM/ESICM/ACCP/ATS/SIS International sepsis definitions conference. *Crit Care Med* 2003; 31:1250–1256
24. Rello J, Rodriguez A, Lisboa T, et al. PIRO Score for community-acquired pneumonia: a new prediction rule for assessment of severity in intensive care unit patients with community-acquired pneumonia. *Crit Care Med* 2009; 37:456–462.
25. Kellum JA, Kong L, Fink MP, Weissfeld LA, Yealy DM, Pinsky MR, Fine J, Krichevsky A, Delude RL, Angus DC; GenIMS Investigators: Understanding the inflammatory cytokine response in pneumonia and sepsis: results of the genetic and inflammatory markers of sepsis (GenIMS) study. *Arch Intern Med* 2007; 167:1655–1663
26. Pifarre R, Falguera M, Vicente-de-Vera C, Nogues A. Characteristics of community-acquired pneumonia in patients with chronic obstructive pulmonary disease. *Respir Med* 2007; 101: 2139–2144
27. Rello J, Rodriguez A, Torres A, Roig J, Sole-Violan J, Garnacho-Montero J, de la Torre MV, Sirvent JM, Bodi M. Implications of COPD in patients admitted to the intensive care unit by community-acquired pneumonia. *Eur Respir J* 2006; 27:1210–1216
28. Brito V, Niederman MS. How can we improve the management and outcome of pneumonia in the elderly. *Eur Respir J* 2008; 32:12–14
29. Kothe H, Bauer T, Marre R, et al. Outcome of community-acquired pneumonia: influence of age, residence status and antimicrobial treatment. *Eur Respir J* 2008; 32:139–146
30. Kee C, Palladino S, Kay I, et al. Feasibiltiy of real-time polymerase chain reactin in whole blood to identify *Streptococcus pneumoniae* in patients with community-acquired pneumonia. *Diagn Microbiol Infect Dis* 2008; 61:72–75
31. Rello J, Lisboa T, Lujan M, et al. Severity of Pneumococcal Pneumonia Associated with Genomic Bacterial Load. *Chest* 2009 [in press]
32. Rello J, Bodi M, Mariscal D, Navarro M, Diaz E, Gallego M, Valles J. Microbiological testing and outcome of patients with severe community-acquired pneumonia. *Chest* 2003; 123:174–180
33. Bodi M, Rodriguez A, Sole-Violan J, et al. Antibiotic prescription for community-acqured pneumonia in the intensive care unit: impact of adherence to IDSA guidelines on survival. *Clin Infect Dis* 2005; 41:1709–1716
34. Restrepo MI, Mortensen EM, Waterer GW, et al. Impact of macrolide therapy on mortality for patients with severe sepsis due to pneumonia. *Eur Respir J* 2009; 33:153–159
35. Annane D, Meduri GU, Marik P. Critical illness related corticosteroid insufficiency and community-acquired pneumonia: back to the future! *Eur Resp J* 2008; 31:1150–1152
36. Dellinger RP, Levy MM, Carlet J, et al. Surviving sepsis campaing. International guidelines for management of severe sepsis and septic shock: 2008 *Intensive Care Med* 2008; 34:17–60

37. Salluh JL, Bozza FA, Soares M, et al. Adrenal response in severe community-acquired pneumonia: impact on outcomes and disease severity. *Chest* 2008; 134:947–954
38. Rodriguez A, Lisboa T, Blot S, et al. Mortality in bacterial community-acquired pneumonia: when antibiotics are not enough. *Intensive Care Med* 2009; 35:430–438.
39. Torres A, Serra-Batlles J, Ferrer A, et al. Severe community-acquired pneumonia. *Am Rev Respir Dis* 1991; 144:312–318

Real-Time PCR in Microbiology: From Diagnosis to Characterization

Malte Book, Lutz Eric Lehmann, Xiang Hong Zhang, and Frank Stueber

1 Introduction

In 1991 the American College of Chest Physicians (ACCP) and the Society of Critical Care Medicine (SCCM) initiated the so-called consensus conference for precise and consistent definitions of the terms "sepsis" and "organ failure" [1]. This conference introduced the term "systemic inflammatory response syndrome (SIRS)" to clinical practice, which was not much appreciated but nevertheless implemented universally in the clinical language. In the following years, knowledge about the interaction of pathogens and human defense systems increased rapidly. However, improvement of the clinical outcome of patients suffering from infection and/or inflammation could not keep up with the simultaneous fundamental improvements in the understanding of the molecular mechanisms. Therefore, in 2001 it was necessary to revive the consensus conference toward three major goals [2]. (a) To review the strength and weakness of current definitions and related conditions. (b) To identify ways of improving the current definitions. (c) To provide methodologies for increasing the accuracy, reliability, and/or clinical utility of the diagnosis of sepsis. In brief, the conclusions of the 2001 International Sepsis Definitions Conference were: (a) Current concepts of sepsis, severe sepsis, and septic shock remain useful to clinicians and researchers. (b) These definitions do not allow precise staging or prognostication of the host response to infection. (c) While SIRS is a useful concept, the diagnostic criteria for SIRS published in 1992 are overly sensitive and nonspecific. (d) An expanded list of signs and symptoms of sepsis may better reflect the clinical response to infection. Despite these results, participants in this conference characterized a major weak point in the current-definition of sepsis: It lacked a precise characterization and staging of patients. A useful staging system stratifies patients according to (a) their baseline risk for an adverse outcome and (b) their potential to respond to the therapy. A prototype for an effective staging system is the "tumor, lymph nodes, metastasis" (TNM) system used in oncology for more than 60 years [3]. In this process the description of the primary tumor itself (T), metastases

M. Book (✉)
University Department of Anaesthesiology and Pain Therapy, Inselspital, CH-3010 Bern, Switzerland
e-mail: Malte.Book@dkf.ubibe.ch

to regional lymph nodes (N), and distant metastases (M) are considered and each domain is graded to denote the extent of pathological involvement. The previously reported conclusions of the 2001 conference are enhancements and modifications of existing concepts. In contrast, the development of a sepsis classification scheme is an innovation. The staging of patients can be performed on the basis of four major variables: predisposition, infection, response, and organ dysfunction. One of the visions of the 2001 consensus conference participants was to establish arrays for the detection of microbial products (lipopolysaccharide [LPS], galactomannan, bacterial DNA) and gene transcription profiles. These detection arrays are crucial for further therapies directed specifically against particular cell wall components or critical receptor constituents.

The relevance of bacterial DNA, in particular, has been under investigation for more than 10 years. Unmethylated CpG dinucleotide motifs are present in prokaryotic cells, whereas in eukaryotic cells CpG motifs are frequently suppressed by methylization [4, 5]. These unmethylated CpG motifs have been identified as potent activators of immune cells [6–8]. In 1997 Sparwasser and coworkers reported on the stimulation of the macrophage cell line ANA-1 by unmethylated CpG motifs that result in fulminant-dose and species-dependant tumor necrosis factor (TNF) release [9]. High CpG concentrations are as sufficient as endotoxin stimulation in the ANA-1 cell line [9]. Moreover, mice that were injected intraperitoneally with DNA from Gram-positive or Gram-negative bacteria showed increased circulating TNF plasma levels [9]. In an ex-vivo experiment, peritoneal macrophages from LPS nonresponder C3H/HeJ mice showed TNF release following DNA, but not due to endotoxin stimulation [9]. These findings demonstrated the potential proinflammatory effect of DNA oligonucleotides, which is not identical to the endotoxin pathway. The effect of these proinflammatory CpG motifs is mediated by the TLR (toll-like receptor) 9 receptor [10].

2
Whole-Blood Culture as Gold Standard for BSI Detection

Sepsis, severe sepsis, and septic shock are common and especially dangerous diseases that have been underestimated in the past. Data acquired by the German SepNet revealed the high prevalence of sepsis in Germany [11]. Bloodstream infections (BSIs) are a major component in the pathogenesis of septic diseases. Weinstein and coworkers detected a mortality rate of about 17% in patients with bacteremia [12]. Moreover, their observation was in accordance with other groups and they presented an appropriate antimicrobial therapy as the most effective way to lower mortality [12–16]. Early detection and adequate treatment of causative pathogens within the first 6–12 h, however, are critical for a favorable outcome in patients with BSI [17–19]. The guidelines for management of severe sepsis and septic shock even recommend calculated antimicrobial therapy within the first hour according to current clinical investigations [20]. Kumar and coworkers showed that from the onset of hypotension in patients presenting with septic shock, each hour of delay in antimicrobial administration was associated with an average 8% decrease in survival rate [21]. A meta-analysis confirmed that inadequate initial antimicrobial therapy increased patients' odds of mortality [22]. In clinical routine practice, Tumbarello and coworkers reported that 43% of the patients suffering from BSI caused by extended spectrum beta lactamase (ESBL)-producing *Escherichia coli* had initially received inadequate antimicrobial therapy [23]. The duration of this inadequate therapy was between 48 and 120 h, with a mean of 72 h [23]. Independent risk factors were unknown BSI source, isolate coresistance to three or more antimicrobials, hospitalization during the 12 months preceding BSI onset, and antimicrobial therapy during the 3 months preceding BSI onset [23]. Inadequate initial antimicrobial therapy was the strongest risk factor for 21-day mortality and significantly increased the length of hospitalization after BSI onset [23].

The first report on a BSI was presented more than a century ago. In 1897 Libman described two children with bloody diarrhea in the course of streptococcal disease [24]. Nine years later he published a series of 700 blood cultures including guidelines on how to process this material [25]. Since then, blood cultures have become an important diagnostic tool, and since the invention of antimicrobial agents they have also been used to test pathogen susceptibility for the therapeutic effect of antibiotics. The protocols for obtaining the blood samples, performing the culturing, and detecting microbial growth have been improved constantly. At present, blood culturing is the gold standard for diagnosis of bacteremia in patients with fever.

In spite of all these improvements, clinicians should still keep in mind the weak points of blood culture as a diagnostic tool. Blood culture typically becomes positive 8–36 h after sampling. The initial empiric therapy can then be adapted based on presumptive bacterial identification suggested by the Gram-stain characteristics. A more precise pathogen identification and susceptibility profile, however, is not available until up to 24–48 h later [15, 26]. The culturing time has to be extended especially when slow-growing organisms such as *Mycobacterium tuberculosis* or fastidious organisms such as *Bartonella spp.* are suspected. In these instances therapy remains empiric and is initiated long before culture results become available. The essential time for the culturing process has not been shortened convincingly in the past 100 years. Today, the need for culturing time appears to be a major impairment of this method. The time from empiric to adapted therapy is long, and for some fatal cases it may have been too long.

The blood culture technique is limited by the low a priori chance of isolating certain pathogens. It has a poor specificity and false-positive rates range from 5 to 50% depending on the methods of collection [12, 27]. Despite optimization of the technique, only 15–25% of positive results can be anticipated. In up to 30% of patients with fever, clear results cannot be obtained at all [28–30]. In particular, blood culture sensitivity for slow-growing and fastidious organisms can be poor. Some organisms that are important causes of community-acquired pneumonia, such as *Legionella pneumophila, Chlamydia pneumoniae,* and *Mycoplasma pneumoniae,* are poorly detectable [31]. The identification of pathogens using the blood culture technique is significantly limited by previously initiated antimicrobial therapy [32–34]. However, an even more common clinical scenario is a patient with signs of systemic infections treated by empiric antimicrobial therapy and recurring episodes of fever. Because of these limitations, researchers and clinicians are motivated to compensate at least partially for the limitations of the blood culture technique and, on the other hand, to establish additional methods to supplement the diagnostic tools for BSIs. In particular, the development of methods that shorten the time period to acquisition of significant results has been identified as an important medical need. Molecular techniques have a potential to fulfill this need [26].

3
Identification of Pathogens in Growth-Positive Blood Cultures

The first detection of microbial components via a DNA probe was made in 1988 by Malouin and coworkers [35]. A ^{32}P-labeled 5-kb *Haemophilus influenzae* DNA fragment detected spotted *H. influenzae* diluted in human serum, urine sputum, or cerebrospinal fluid [35]. In 1991 Davis and coworkers reported the detection of *Staphylococcus aureus, Streptococcus pneumoniae, E. coli, H. influenzae, Enterococcus sp.*, and *S. agalactiae* in blood cultures by using a chemiluminescent DNA probe [36]. Subsequently, nucleic acid-based diagnostic systems, including polymerase chain reaction (PCR) methods as well as the application of DNA and RNA probes, have proven to be sensitive techniques for a more rapid detection and specific identification of pathogens involved in BSI [37–42]. Moreover, these methods are widely used to decrease laboratory turnaround times so that results can be available to the clinician at an earlier stage. The currently used techniques for identification of pathogens in growth-positive blood cultures can de divided into hybridization-based and amplification-based techniques.

The hybridization-based approach consists of chemiluminescence-labeled DNA probes to target ribosomal 16s or 18s DNA (rDNA). They complement the sequence of small-subunit rRNA and form a duplex molecule if the target sequence is present. The resulting labeled duplex molecule can then be detected. These assays allow for the identification of many pathogens within 60 min at the level of the genus, species, or both, depending on the matrices used [43]. Polymicrobial infections can be identified by the simultaneous detection of two different chemiluminescence patterns or can be suspected by comparing the strengths of genus-specific or species-specific probe signals with the signal obtained using an all-bacteria probe.

The hybridization-based approach is a sensitive and specific technique that merits further evaluation in clinical practice. Future advancement with miniaturization will provide the opportunity for parallel species testing and detection of resistance genes and multibacterial infections.

The so-called FISH (fluorescence in situ hybridization) technique uses slides of growth-positive cultures, in which cells are permeabilized and hybridized with fluorochrome-labeled oligonucleotide probes targeted to rRNA. Fluorescence is the result of the binding of the oligonucleotide probe to target RNA and is visualized by microscopy. FISH allows identification within 2.5 h of more than 95% of most bacteria and yeasts commonly found in blood [39–44].

The amplification of bacterial components by real-time PCR from growth-positive blood cultures is the most common method. The anticoagulant sodium polyanetholesulfonate used in blood cultures has to be antagonized first by use of guanidine hydrochloride-benzyl alcohol DNA extraction [45]. Addition of bovine serum albumin results in further prevention of inhibitory effects [46]. The fast detection of resistance genes, e.g., the macA-gene in *Staphylococcus* and vanA/vanB in *Enterococcus*, is widely used today in clinical routine approaches [47]. It must be mentioned that PCR methods are more complex and their technical preconditions exceed those of other techniques. This makes the PCR method more expensive.

Theoretically, PCR detection allows the confirmation of only a few pathogen colony-forming units (CFUs). This superior sensitivity is foiled by the fact that the PCR method

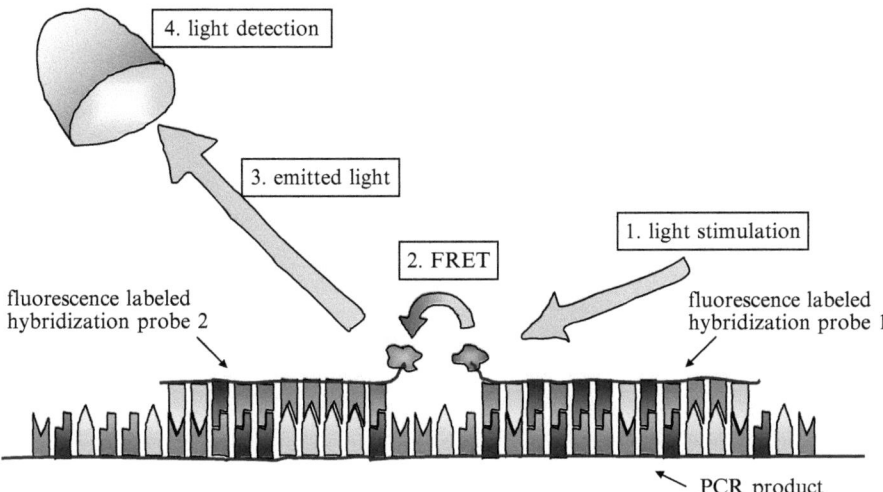

Fig. 1 Schematic picture of two fluorescence-labeled hybridization probes binding specifically to the PCR product. In the heating phase the melting temperature can be determined by the repeated cycle of: (1) Light stimulation of the hybridized probe 1. (2) Fluorescence resonance energy transfer (FRET) from probe 1 to probe 2. (3) Light emission of hybridization probe 2, which (4) will de detected by the PCR device. The melting of one probe results in the immediate termination of FRET which rules out the further detection of light

starts after a positive blood culture signal is detectable, which indicates a high pathogen concentration. Therefore, PCR is not used to detect low pathogen concentrations in this setting. The reasonable use of PCR from growth-positive blood cultures is limited to a few diagnostic indications: identification of pathogens with long generation times, otherwise slow-growing times, or difficulties in culturing. Moreover, it may be useful in the diagnosis of very rare pathogens such as *Pasteurella pneumotropica*, *Moraxella atlantae*, or *Tsukamurella species* [48].

Cleven and coworkers presented alternative techniques for pathogen detection following positive blood culture results. This group worked with an array technique that identifies cultured pathogens and specific resistance genes [49]. In this first study, *S. aureus*, *E. coli*, and *Pseudomonas aeruginosa* were detected by species-specific gene probes spotted on a DNA microarray. In addition, resistance genes were tested and the phenotypic antibiotic resistance showed a large correlation to the genotypic one [49].

4
Direct PCR Detection

The first direct detection of pathogens from whole blood by using the PCR technique was reported in 1993 by Song and coworkers. Two pairs of oligonucleotide primers were designed for the amplification of a 343-bp fragment of the flagellin gene of *Salmonella typhi* in patients with typhoid fever [50]. By using a nested PCR technique, ten organisms of *S. typhi* were detected [50]. The PCR products were detected by agarose gel electrophoresis followed by radioactive-labeled Southern blot hybridization [50]. In this study with limited sample size, 11 of 12 patients with typhoid fever that was confirmed by blood culture were positive for the *S. typhi* flagellin DNA fragment [50]. Shortly after, Iralu and colleagues reported on the PCR detection of *Mycobacterium avium* DNA from purified and lysed peripheral blood mononuclear cells [51]. PCR results in this form were analyzed by subsequent radioactive-labeled hybridization probes. This investigation that also had a limited sample size reported a sensitivity of 80% [51].

The main advantage of these PCR techniques is the considerable reduction of time, which could result in faster application of an adequate antimicrobial therapy to sepsis patients. PCR methods for the single detection of *M. tuberculosis, E. coli, Neisseria meningitidis,* and *S. pneumoniae* have been published [52–58]. However, in a clinical setting with a septic patient in the emergency room, it is not feasible to use a PCR-based diagnostic procedure employing several PCR reactions which specifically test for each pathogen. The detection of universal bacterial components in the blood, the so-called broad range or universal PCR, was a considerable advancement of the existing single-pathogen-specific approach. Amplification of 16s or 23s rRNA that is present in all bacteria is able to indicate the presence of bacterial components in the blood. A similar method has been reported to be successful in fungi detection [59]. Further identification of the amplicons by capillary sequencing analysis, pyrosequencing, or hybridization with specific probes has been used to discriminate between pathogens [60, 61].

As revealed in recent studies, about 20–25 pathogen species account for more than 90% of all detected nosocomial pathogens in BSIs [62]. Furthermore, methodological improvements in PCR technology now enable the detection of the most common pathogens in one PCR run. This so-called multiplex PCR works with a variety of specific primers. Therefore, the simultaneous detection of a previously defined pathogen panel is possible. Corless and coworkers established a PCR-based detection method of the three most common causes of meningitis and septicemia in children (*N. meningitidis, H. influenzae,* and *S. pneumoniae*) in an assay from cerebrospinal fluid, plasma, serum, and whole blood [63]. In addition, with this investigation they detected infections that had not been discovered by culturing techniques.

In 2002 Klaschik and coworkers reported on the discrimination between 17 Gram-positive and Gram-negative bacteria in variable human body fluids. The amplification was performed by a highly conserved part of the 16s DNA with one primer pair for 17 organisms in a real-time PCR. The discrimination between Gram-positive and -negative bacteria was made by labeled hybridization probes that allowed a completely regular classification of Gram status [64]. The overall time needed for this analysis was about 3 h. Current investigations expand the number of pathogens that are detectable in parallel by the use of multiplex PCR technique. The detection of up to 25 bacterial and fungal pathogens in one PCR reaction was reported in 2007 [65]. It is important that, in principle, PCR allows the detection of bacterial components even if there is no chance for pathogen proliferation and an antimicrobial therapy is useless. At present, it is unclear whether this fact should be assessed as an advantage or as a disadvantage. On the one hand, the detection of such proinflammatory nucleotides might enable specific therapy in the future according to the visions of the 2001 consensus conference participants. On the other hand, the discrimination of vital from nonvital components is crucial for the initiation of antimicrobial therapy in daily routine.

5
Implementation of Real-Time PCR Pathogen Detection in Clinical Practice

To date, real-time PCR is used increasingly for pathogen detection. The diagnosis of pneumococcal infection is difficult. The presence of *Streptococcus pneumoniae* in the nasopharynx gives information about colonization but not about infection, and the blood culture detection method is limited by its poor sensitivity of 10 to 30% [66]. In a model with transnasally infected mice, the blood culture method was compared with a real-time PCR assay targeting the autolysin (*lytA*) and pneumococcal surface adhesion (*psaA*) genes. After infection, mice were treated with ceftriaxone prior to PCR and blood culture sampling. Blood culture results following administration of the antimicrobial agent were remarkably poor. Twenty-four hours after infection and 2–6 h after ceftriaxone administration, 100% of blood cultures in 16 mice were negative [67]. However, in this group 81% of real-time PCR results indicated bacterial components in the blood detected by the *psaA* gene [67]. The *lytA* detection yielded 88% positive results in this group [67]. These data highlight the difference between the two methods. Whereas blood culturing detects vital pathogens, PCR techniques detect bacterial components, independently of vitality.

Beside the results of murine assays, real-time PCR tests for pneumococcal infections have also proven their applicability in patients. The incidence of pneumococcal parapneumonic empyema is increasing. Especially in children, about 0.6% of all pneumonias progress to empyema. This results in a prevalence of 3.3 affected children per 100,000 [68]. Identification of the pathogen by culturing methods is hampered by their low sensitivity. In 8% of pleural fluids and in less than 10% of blood specimens, the pathogen was identified by culturing methods [69, 70]. Tarrago and coworkers established a real-time PCR approach to detect the pneumococcal *wzg* gene. Using this method, 175 strains representing 35 serotypes were identified with a minimum of 12–24 fg of DNA [71]. The reevaluation of 88 culture-negative samples with real-time PCR resulted in the identification of pneumococcal DNA in 88% of samples [71]. The parallel determination of infection and resistance pattern has also been investigated in *Streptococcus pneumoniae*. By using a duplex real-time PCR reaction, Harris and coworkers detected the *S. pneumoniae lytA* gene and the penicillin-binding protein 2b (pbp2b) gene occurring in penicillin-susceptible organisms in parallel. All organisms that showed an MIC > 1.0 mg L^{-1} were pbp2b real-time PCR negative [72]. Twelve isolates were penicillin susceptible (MICs of < or = 0.06 mg L^{-1}) and pbp2b real-time PCR positive [72]. In summary, the presented data indicate the potential of resistance testing by using real-time PCR in humans.

The increasing frequency of BSI caused by methicillin-resistant *Staphylococcus aureus* (MRSA) was recognized as a serious medical problem in the late 1980s [73, 74]. The preliminary blood culture diagnosis "Gram-positive cocci, possibly Staphylococcus" in critically ill patients with signs of BSIs resulted frequently in the administration of vancomycin in these patients. However, only in a fraction of these isolates was the diagnosis of MRSA confirmed. An evaluation of 19 Canadian intensive care units (ICUs) found an MRSA frequency of 22.3% in all *Staphylococcus aureus* isolates [75]. The subsequent widespread use of vancomycin is partially responsible for the increasing frequency of vancomycin-resistant enterococci (VRE) infections in critically ill patients [76, 77]. Therefore, it is very important to save time in the diagnosis of MRSA BSIs. Real-time PCR methods have been tested to fulfill this need. The commercial kit BD GeneOhm StaphSR assay (BD GeneOhm, San Diego, CA) was designed for the differentiation between methicillin-susceptible *Staphylococcus aureus* (MSSA) and MRSA. It is a real-time PCR assay that works with different sets of primers in parallel as a multiplex PCR. Stamper and coworkers tested the clinical practicability of this system and found excellent sensitivity in the discrimination between MSSA and MRSA [78]. However, this method started with the detection of a positive blood culture. Therefore, the culturing time cannot be reduced by this kit. In the field of experimental tests a much more rapid detection of MRSA was described in 2004 by Huletski and coworkers. In a multiplex PCR containing five pairs of primers, the detection of MRSA directly from nonsterile clinical specimens was possible in less than 1 h [79]. The sensitivity of this assay was 98.7%; false-positive MRSA detection was reported in 4.6% of cases [79]. Thomas and coworkers described an alternative approach with a duplex PCR reaction targeting the species-specific *nuc* gene and the *mecA* gene encoding methicillin resistance [80]. A comparison of two molecular real-time PCR methods with two selective MRSA agars illustrated advantages and disadvantages for the different methods [81]. Detailed product descriptions are available in the original publication [81]. Table 1 gives an overview of the authors' main findings in 200 consecutive high-risk patients.

For defined questions, real-time PCR expanded the panel of diagnostic tools in an effective way. However, the future challenge is pathogen detection without a limited number of suspects.

Table 1 Comparison of two molecular real-time PCR methods and two agars for MRSA detection [81]

Detection method	Sensitivity (%)	Specificity (%)	Processing time[a] (min)	Total cost[b] ($)	Results (h)
Molecular detection					
Kit 1	86	98	15	53.60	2
Kit 2	84	90	5	11.10	3
Selective agars @ 24 h					
Agar 1	62	100	10	9.80	24–48
Agar 2	84	99	10	9.50	24–48
Selective agars @ 48 h					
Agar 1	89	93	–	–	–
Agar 2	91	70	–	–	–

[a] Processing time is the hands-on time required by the scientist remunerated at $33.68 per hour

[b] Total cost = cost per test + consumable/reagents cost + (processing time×33.68) [Australian dollars]

6
Rapid Detection and Differentiation of 25 Bacterial and Fungal Pathogens by Multiplex Real-Time PCR from Whole Blood

This method was reported by Lehmann and coworkers in 2008 [65]. In contrast to other approaches, it started with DNA preparation from whole blood. The advantage of the technique is the detection of bacterial cells or DNA already incorporated in macrophages. The pathogens included in this test are displayed in Table 2.

Initially, 3 ml whole blood is collected in a potassium-ethylenediaminetetraacetic acid (K-EDTA) container without preculturing. The whole-blood samples and the set-up of the PCR reaction have to be prepared in a laminar flow box to minimize the risk of workflow contamination. In addition, the use of high-quality DNA-free reagents and plasticware is an essential precondition for this test. The reaction starts with the parallel amplification of Gram-positive bacteria, Gram-negative bacteria, and fungi in three parallel reactions. Primers for bacterial amplification are located between the 16S and the 23S ribosomal DNA sequences and fungal primers are located between the 18S and 5.8S ribosomal sequences. Discrimination between the different pathogens is made by specific hybridization probes that anneal to the PCR products. Following light stimulation of the first hybridization probe, the light energy passes to the second probe, which is bonded in direct proximity, by fluorescence resonance energy transfer (FRET). This second probe emits a light signal that can be detected by the PCR device. This sequence is displayed schematically in Fig. 1.

Depending on the length and the sequence of the probes as well as the grade of matching to the target, a melting temperature is known for each probe – target complex. At this temperature the probes separate from the PCR target and the energy transfer and light emission stops. Therefore, the temperature is increased continuously by 0.1 °C per second, and the temperature at which the detectable light emission stops characterizes the melting temperature. The emitted light can be detected in four different wavelengths (610, 640, 670

Table 2 Twenty-five detectable pathogens included in the real-time PCR whole-blood test

Gram-negative	Gram-positive	Fungi
Escherichia coli	*Staphylococcus aureus*	*Candida albicans*
Klebsiella (pneumoniae/ oxytoca)	CoNS	*Candida tropicalis*
Serratia marcescens	*Streptococcus pneumoniae*	*Candida parapsilosis*
Enterobacter (cloacae/ aerogenes)	*Streptococcus spp.*	*Candida krusei*
Proteus mirabilis	*Enterococcus faecium*	*Candida glabrata*
Pseudomonas aeruginosa	*Enterococcus faecalis*	*Aspergillus fumigatus*
Acinetobacter baumannii	–	–
Stenotrophomonas maltophilia	–	–

and 705 nm), which in combination with the temperature allow the characterization of different pathogens. The complete protocol needs less than 6 h for the whole workflow, which is an enormous saving of time compared to the blood culturing methods. To increase analytical sensitivity, the internal transcribed spacer (ITS) region was selected as the target region for bacterial (16S–23S) and fungal (18S–5.8S) species identification. The ITS region offers higher analytical sensitivity compared to single-copy targets since it is present in multiple operons in the genomes of bacteria and fungi [82]. Moreover, the ITS region is more species-specific compared to the conserved rDNA genomic region and, therefore, is more suitable for species differentiation [83]. The sensitivity of this real-time PCR method depends on the pathogen. One hundred CFUs per milliliter were detected in a series with different pathogens in each sample [65]. In serial experiments performed on EDTA-blood samples spiked with different concentrations of bacterial and fungal reference organisms, hit rates of 70–100% were achieved for 23 of 25 organisms with 30 CFU mL^{-1} and for 15 of 25 organisms with 3 CFU mL^{-1} [65]. The sensitivity of pathogen detection in whole-blood cultures was described to be higher with 1–30 CFU mL^{-1} [84, 85]. However, the overall sensitivity (number of detected isolates/number of isolates tested) was reported to be 98.8%, with an overall accuracy of 98.8% (number of correctly detected isolates/number of isolates detected) in the investigation by Lehmann [65].

7
Contamination Is a Serious Problem for PCR Amplification Techniques

Ribosomal RNA has been considered as a target sequence for pathogen detection since the 1980s. As the detectability of variable or conserved rRNA structures by labeled oligonucleotides is limited, several researchers have taken the approach to amplify these regions by the currently emerging PCR technique [86–89]. Contamination by tiny amounts of PCR products carrying from one reaction to the other is a well-known cause of false-positive results [90]. The PCR detection of bacterial rDNA is complicated by the prevalently existing contamination of PCR reagents by any kind of eubacterial DNA. In particular, *Taq* polymerase is frequently contaminated by bacterial DNA [91–93]. It has been reported that in non-decontaminated PCR assays using universal primers, background levels of up to 1,000 copies of contaminating *E. coli* DNA can be present, thereby impairing the analytical sensitivity of such assays [94]. This amount of contaminated DNA and the high frequency of contaminated PCR reagents are not acceptable in a method with the aim of supporting blood culture techniques in which a single vital organism is theoretically detectable. The treatment of the PCR reagents with 8-methoxypsoralen and UV irradiation was reported to be useful for reagent decontamination [95, 96]. However, damaging the *Taq* polymerase was described as a major limitation of this method [97]. Meier and coworkers established a protocol in 1992 that is sufficient for reagent decontamination by the use of 8-methoxypsoralen and long-wave UV light irradiation [94]. In 2002 Klaschik and colleagues described the advantage of decontamination approaches adjusted for use with real-time PCR techniques. They tested the following in detail: (a) DNAse treatment of PCR reagents; (b) UV irradiation for nicking contaminating genomic DNA; (c) treatment with 8-methoxypsoralen in combination with long-wave UV light to render contaminating DNA unamplifiable; and (d) digestion with restriction endonuclease to remove contaminating DNA [98]. Most of the decontamination procedures for PCR failed to eliminate the contaminating bacterial DNA. Furthermore, all of the decontamination procedures led to degradation of the *Taq* polymerases used in real-time PCRs either by UV light or by heat. Even the most efficient procedure, DNAse decontamination, compromised the polymerase, mainly through the long heat inactivation step for the DNAse. All decontamination methods for PCR are time consuming and bring the possibility of carrying new contamination into the reaction mixture. To detect low copy numbers of bacterial DNA in clinical specimens, the target DNA must be differentiated from contaminating, exogenous bacterial DNA. Therefore, clean working conditions are essential and decontamination with DNAse is promising, but above all, it is necessary to have PCR reagents that are free of nucleic acids [63, 98]. These methods represent a major improvement, as conventional non-decontaminated PCR reagents usually show a background threshold of between 500 and 1,000 copies of bacterial target DNA/reaction [94, 98]. It is an interesting fact that *Taq* DNA polymerase has a high affinity for DNA [92], which probably makes it impossible to completely eliminate contaminating DNA, since the polymerase itself always protects small amounts of such DNA against decontamination.

8
The Spectrum of Multiplex Real-Time PCR Diagnostic Products Is Expanding

8.1
Seeplex System by Seegene

This newly available test starts with the screening of 64 pathogens that might cause sepsis. As a result, three Gram-positive groups, two Gram-negative groups, and one fungi group including 22, 24, two, five, five, and six pathogens, respectively, are detectable. Results are available within 5 h and the test can be performed from whole blood, cerebrospinal fluid, blood cultures, urine, and other body fluids. The results of the screening step are visualized by an auto-electrophoresis system. The facultative sepsis ID test reveals 26 pathogens distributed in five groups. This second step is practicable with identical specimens as the first part. In addition the resistance genes *mecA, vanA,* and *vanB* are detectable in the second multiplex PCR reaction. In the company's product presentation there is no information concerning the primer binding sites. Moreover, precise values for sensitivity and specificity are not mentioned. No information about the problem of contamination is available. The search term "seeplex + sepsis" in the PubMed database resulted in one publication on a kit for the detection of respiratory viruses. This test kit is for research use only and is not available in the United States.

8.2
VYOO System by Sirs-Lab

This test detects 34 bacterial, six fungal species, and five resistance genes. The detectable resistance genes are: *vanA, vanB, vanC, blaSHV,* and *mecA*. Product information mentions that these 40 pathogens encompass 99% of all sepsis-relevant pathogens. After the cell lyses, a concentration step of the pathogen DNA is performed by a column set. This step is essential for increasing the sensitivity of downstream PCR protocols and for removing human background DNA. Pathogens are detected by a multiplex PCR reaction and results are visualized by gel electrophoresis. The results of the test are available after 8 h. The product information presents a study with 46 patients. The conclusion is that this test is more specific and more sensitive than the blood culture method. A PubMed search of "vyoo + sepsis" does not result in any hit. The technical note of the VYOO test explains that this tool is allowed for research use only. However, the CE-IVD (Conformité Européene-in vitro-diagnostic) mark is pictured on the company's VYOO® Web site. This might be a hint of a planned or recently successful application for this European mark. There is no detailed information about the problem of contamination or highly purified reagents.

8.3
Sepsitest System by Molzym

This test is designed to detect Gram-positive and Gram-negative bacteria as well as fungi by the use of universal rDNA primers. Similar to the previous test, in Sepsitest human DNA is removed after selective human cell lyses. As for other PCR-based tests, contamination is a serious problem for preserving high sensitivity. Therefore, traces of artificial DNA are removed prior to customer use. This allows the detection of 40 *S. aureus* CFUs per milliliter blood. The PCR reaction can be set up in different PCR devices and the PCR products have to be sequenced for identification, which results in a total time needed of about 6 h and in a high number of detectable pathogens. More than 345 bacteria and fungi are identifiable. In the product description a preliminary investigation for specificity and sensitivity quantification is presented. In this comparison of blood culture and Sepsitest, 21 patients suffering from SIRS are included. The investigation found eight positive blood culture results and seven positive Sepsitest results. This test is not biased by free DNA that has been present, for example, due to bacteria lysis by phagocytes. The DNA isolation technology leads exclusively to material released by intact living cells. The PubMed query "sepsitest + sepsis" also does not result in any hit. This test can be used for therapy monitoring outside the United States because it received CE-IVD marking according to the European in vitro diagnostic directive EN 98/79/EG.

8.4
LightCycler SeptiFast Test System by Roche

This system is based on the publication by Lehmann and coworkers, which was discussed previously in this in this chapter. Briefly, the main specifications are: It is a real-time PCR-based system for the identification of 25 pathogens (nine Gram-positive, nine Gram-negative, and seven fungi). It is a multiplex PCR reaction, and pathogen identification is performed by labeled hybridization probes. This test is marked CE-IVD according to the European directives. A PubMed search for "septifast + sepsis" yielded three hits [99–101].

8.5
Which One Is the Best?

All available test systems lack the scientific evidence that sepsis patients benefit from the test results. Three of these systems are very new and one system has been available since 2006. The sensitivity and specificity of these tests have to be determined in large multi-center trials with a calculated sample size for adequate power. Finally, it should be noted whether the PCR test data result in a modification of the antimicrobial therapy. The technical needs of the four kits are different. The existing infrastructure in the microbiology department and primarily the skills of the technicians should be taken into account. Otherwise the learning curve of a team that is not aware of the susceptibility for contamination in the real-time PCR setting will be quite long. Three of the four available systems are limited to a number of up to 34 detectable pathogens. Since the pathogen spectrum and the frequency of single pathogens may be different in distinct ICUs, a test with a limited number of pathogens might be ineffective. Moreover, only two of the systems are admitted as a diagnostic tool, whereas the other two are allowed for research use only.

9
Conclusion

The diagnosis and quickest possible therapy of BSIs is crucial for sepsis patients. Pathogen detection by blood culturing was established more than 100 years ago, and the disadvantage of the long times demanded has not been solved effectively. In particular, early initiation of an adequate antimicrobial therapy for BSI is crucial for the prognosis, since an inadequate initial antimicrobial therapy increases the patients' odds of mortality. In principle, two methods may support the blood culture results: First, pathogen detection by amplification or hybridization from cultured specimens. Because the culturing step is necessary, this procedure does not reduce the time needed for the blood culture method considerably. Second, the direct detection of pathogens in human specimens by PCR amplification. To date, four different kits based on the PCR amplification of pathogen components are available and two of them are admitted for diagnosis in patients, whereas the other two are for research use only.

In comparisons between broad-range PCR and blood culture methods, bacterial DNA was detected in more than 25% of culture-negative blood samples from neutropenic patients with fever during chemotherapy or bone marrow transplantation, from febrile adult patients in intensive care, and from critically ill surgical patients after multiple trauma, major operation, or solid-organ transplantation [102–105]. How should one interpret a positive PCR result with a parallel negative blood culture result? Potentially, the result can be false positive due to contamination of the PCR reagents. On the other hand, it might be correct and the blood culture may have failed because of fastidious microorganisms, microorganisms that grow poorly, or owing to previous use of antibiotics. A direct comparison of this PCR method with the blood culture method is difficult because blood culture is the gold standard in BSI diagnosis. Therefore, the findings of comparative studies have to be evaluated accurately. A sign of a true-positive PCR result with a negative blood culture result could be:

(a) The detection of the pathogen in a previous or subsequent blood culture. (b) The positive culturing of the pathogen from a normally sterile body fluid.

The two main advantages of PCR-based pathogen detection are, first, the considerable saving of time in comparison to blood culture. Second, PCR-based methods have the potential to improve the sensitivity of the diagnosis of BSIs. Moreover, the complete workflow can be performed within 6–8 h. Therefore, theoretically, PCR-based pathogen detection may save lives by enabling earlier adequate antimicrobial therapy in some patients. This hypothesis seems to be in accordance with the investigation from Kumar, who reported an average 8% decrease in survival rate per hour from the beginning of hypotension in patients with septic shock [21] and the meta-analysis by Kuti [22].

These important benefits have to be seen alongside some impairments of this method. Currently, the number of detectable pathogens is limited. The method established by Lehmann and coworkers allows the detection of 25 pathogens in three parallel real-time PCR reactions. Other kits offering up to 34 parallel pathogen detections are available. The inclusion of more, even clinically infrequent, pathogens can be realized by increasing the number of parallel reactions. However, this would be at the expense of simplicity and practicability. Only the commercially available Sepsitest kit allows the detection of 345 pathogens with the limitation of a necessary subsequent sequencing reaction. Further technical developments in the field of multiplex PCR reactions may extend the possible applications to include uncommon pathogens. Furthermore, the testing of antimicrobial drug resistance consists virtually in blood culturing with supplementary pharmaceuticals. In contrast, PCR-based testing for selected resistance genes is limited in number and is as expensive, time consuming, and complex as pathogen detection itself [49]. Another crucial issue is the PCR method's susceptibility to contaminations. It has been previously reported that in non-decontaminated PCR assays using universal primers, background levels of up to 1,000 copies of contaminating *E. coli* DNA can be present, thereby impairing the analytical sensitivity and specificity of such assays [94]. Such nonspecific signals may arise due to contaminations from environmental microorganisms or by bacterial contamination of PCR ingredients. To avoid nonspecific signals, and to increase analytical sensitivity, high-quality PCR reagents that are free of bacterial or fungal DNA contamination must be used according to suggestions recently discussed in the scientific literature [106, 98]. Furthermore, a positive and negative control and a full process control should be implemented in every run of a PCR-based pathogen detection method. Moreover, the source of the detected pathogen DNA needs further consideration. This DNA may be released from lysed vital organisms. In this case the PCR results would reflect the existence of vital pathogens in the bloodstream and can be interpreted as an actual threat. However, detectable DNA might be derived from lysed macrophages that incorporated the pathogen previously. In this case antimicrobial therapy is too late. Finally, bacteremia has been reported to have occurred consecutively to tooth brushing in 1974, using the blood culture method [107]. This finding has also been confirmed by PCR-supported methods [108]. Therefore, DNA detection in critically ill patients might be interfered by oral hygiene activities as tooth brushing in the ICU. The pathogenetic meaning of this kind of transient bacteremia or transient prevalence of bacterial DNA in the bloodstream of healthy individuals as well as in critically ill patients is unknown. In this regard the Sepsitest might offer interesting results because only DNA from directly lysed vital pathogens is amplified and subsequently detected. However, the assessment of the clinical effect of circulating CpG motifs is still under discussion. It is possible that even the detection of these unmethylated motifs becomes important for future diagnosis or therapy.

In summary, the advancements in the detection and characterization of BSIs are fast paced. Real-time PCR-based clinical findings should be evaluated in clinical investigations and, even more importantly, the potential benefit for critically ill patients with suspected BSIs should be estimated. Currently, supplementing the gold standard method by PCR-based methods might be advantageous.

A promising perspective for the future is the advancement of quantitative real-time PCR techniques. In the field of viral diseases the quantification of DNA is established for diagnosing and monitoring of disease progress [109–112]. In contrast, the field of bacterial DNA quantification is not yet implemented to clinical routine, but it is under intensive research. The first reports described patients with meningococcal sepsis or meningitis in whom meningococcal load correlated well with severity of disease. The quantities of DNA detected ranged between 2.2×10^4 and 1.6×10^8 copies of DNA per milliliter blood [113, 114].

Abbreviations

ACCP	American College of Chest Physicians
BSI	Bloodstream infection
CE-IVD	Conformité Européene-in vitro-diagnostic
CFU	Colony-forming unit
ESBL	Extended spectrum beta-lactamase
FISH	Fluorescence in situ hybridization
FRET	Fluorescence resonance energy transfer
ICU	Intensive care unit
ITS	Internal transcribed spacer
K-EDTA	Potassium-ethylenediaminetetraacetic acid
LPS	Lipopolysaccharide
MRSA	Methicillin-resistant *Staphylococcus aureus*
MSSA	Methicillin-susceptible *Staphylococcus aureus*
PCR	Polymerase chain reaction
SCCM	Society of critical care medicine
SIRS	Systemic inflammatory response syndrome
TLR	Toll-like receptor
TNF	Tumor necrosis factor
TNM	Tumor, lymph nodes, metastasis
VRE	Vancomycin-resistant enterococci

References

1. American College of Chest Physicians/Society of Critical Care Medicine Consensus Conference: definitions for sepsis and organ failure and guidelines for the use of innovative therapies in sepsis (1992) Crit Care Med 20(6):864–874
2. Levy MM, Fink MP, Marshall JC et al. (2003) 2001 SCCM/ESICM/ACCP/ATS/SIS International Sepsis Definitions Conference. Crit Care Med 31(4):1250–1256

3. Denoix P (1946) Enquete permanent dans les centres anticancereaux. Bull Inst Natl Hyg 1(1):70–75
4. Bird AP (1986) CpG-rich islands and the function of DNA methylation. Nature 321(6067):209–213
5. Sutter D, Doerfler W (1980) Methylation of integrated adenovirus type 12 DNA sequences in transformed cells is inversely correlated with viral gene expression. Proc Natl Acad Sci U S A 77(1):253–256
6. Yamamoto S, Yamamoto T, Kataoka T et al. (1992) Unique palindromic sequences in synthetic oligonucleotides are required to induce IFN [correction of INF] and augment IFN-mediated [correction of INF] natural killer activity. J Immunol 148(12):4072–4076
7. Krieg AM, Yi AK, Matson S et al. (1995) CpG motifs in bacterial DNA trigger direct B-cell activation. Nature 374(6522):546–549
8. Pisetsky DS (1996) Immune activation by bacterial DNA: a new genetic code. Immunity 5(4):303–310
9. Sparwasser T, Miethke T, Lipford G et al. (1997) Bacterial DNA causes septic shock. Nature 386(6623):336–337
10. Hemmi H, Takeuchi O, Kawai T et al. (2000) A toll-like receptor recognizes bacterial DNA. Nature 408(6813):740–745
11. Engel C, Brunkhorst FM, Bone HG et al. (2007) Epidemiology of sepsis in Germany: results from a national prospective multicenter study. Intensive Care Med 33(4):606–618
12. Weinstein MP, Towns ML, Quartey SM et al. (1997) The clinical significance of positive blood cultures in the 1990s: a prospective comprehensive evaluation of the microbiology, epidemiology, and outcome of bacteremia and fungemia in adults. Clin Infect Dis 24(4):584–602
13. Leibovici L, Shraga I, Drucker M et al. (1998) The benefit of appropriate empirical antibiotic treatment in patients with bloodstream infection. J Int Med 244(5):379–386
14. Kollef MH (2000) Inadequate antimicrobial treatment: an important determinant of outcome for hospitalized patients. Clin Infect Dis 31(Suppl 4):S131–S138
15. Harbarth S, Garbino J, Pugin J et al. (2003) Inappropriate initial antimicrobial therapy and its effect on survival in a clinical trial of immunomodulating therapy for severe sepsis. Am J Med 115(7):529–535
16. Valles J, Rello J, Ochagavia A et al. (2003) Community-acquired bloodstream infection in critically ill adult patients: impact of shock and inappropriate antibiotic therapy on survival. Chest 123(5):1615–1624
17. Ibrahim EH, Sherman G, Ward S et al. (2000) The influence of inadequate antimicrobial treatment of bloodstream infections on patient outcomes in the ICU setting. Chest 118(1): 146–155
18. Morrell M, Fraser VJ, Kollef MH (2005) Delaying the empiric treatment of candida bloodstream infection until positive blood culture results are obtained: a potential risk factor for hospital mortality. Antimicrob Agents Chemother 49(9):3640–3645
19. Garnacho-Montero J, Garcia-Garmendia JL, Barrero-Almodovar A et al. (2003) Impact of adequate empirical antibiotic therapy on the outcome of patients admitted to the intensive care unit with sepsis. Crit Care Med 31(12):2742–2751
20. Dellinger RP, Carlet JM, Masur H et al. (2004) Surviving sepsis campaign guidelines for management of severe sepsis and septic shock. Crit Care Med 32(3):858–873
21. Kumar A, Roberts D, Wood KE et al. (2006) Duration of hypotension before initiation of effective antimicrobial therapy is the critical determinant of survival in human septic shock. Crit Care Med 34(6):1589–1596
22. Kuti EL, Patel AA, Coleman CI (2008) Impact of inappropriate antibiotic therapy on mortality in patients with ventilator-associated pneumonia and blood stream infection: a meta-analysis. J Crit Care 23(1):91–100

23. Tumbarello M, Sali M, Trecarichi EM et al. (2008) Bloodstream infections caused by extended-spectrum-beta-lactamase- producing *Escherichia coli*: risk factors for inadequate initial antimicrobial therapy. Antimicrob Agents Chemother 52(9):3244–3252
24. Libman E (1897) Weitere Mitteilungen über die Streptokokken-enteritis bei Säuglingen. Zentralbl Bakteriol XXII:376
25. Libman E (1906) On some experiences with blood-cultures in the study of bacterial infections. Johns Hopkins Hosp Bull 17:215–228
26. Struelens MJ, de MR (2001) The emerging power of molecular diagnostics: towards improved management of life-threatening infection. Intensive Care Med 27(11):1696–1698
27. Bates DW, Cook EF, Goldman L et al. (1990) Predicting bacteremia in hospitalized patients. A prospectively validated model. Ann Int Med 113(7):495–500
28. Alberti C, Brun-Buisson C, Burchardi H et al. (2002) Epidemiology of sepsis and infection in ICU patients from an international multicentre cohort study. Intensive Care Med 28(2):108–121
29. Washington JA (1987) The microbiological diagnosis of infective endocarditis. J Antimicrob Chemother 20(Suppl A):29–39
30. Vincent JL, Bihari DJ, Suter PM et al. (1995) The prevalence of nosocomial infection in intensive care units in Europe. Results of the European Prevalence of Infection in Intensive Care (EPIC) Study. EPIC International Advisory Committee. JAMA 274(8):639–644
31. Socan M, Marinic-Fiser N, Kraigher A et al. (1999) Microbial aetiology of community-acquired pneumonia in hospitalised patients. Eur J Clin Microbiol Infect Dis 18(11):777–782
32. McKenzie R, Reimer LG (1987) Effect of antimicrobials on blood cultures in endocarditis. Diagn Microbiol Infect Dis 8(3):165–172
33. Glerant JC, Hellmuth D, Schmit JL et al. (1999) Utility of blood cultures in community-acquired pneumonia requiring hospitalization: influence of antibiotic treatment before admission. Respir Med 93(3):208–212
34. Serody JS, Berrey MM, Albritton K et al. (2000) Utility of obtaining blood cultures in febrile neutropenic patients undergoing bone marrow transplantation. Bone Marrow Transpl 26(5):533–538
35. Malouin F, Bryan LE, Shewciw P et al. (1988) DNA probe technology for rapid detection of *Haemophilus influenzae* in clinical specimens. J Clin Microbiol 26(10):2132–2138
36. Davis TE, Fuller DD (1991) Direct identification of bacterial isolates in blood cultures by using a DNA probe. J Clin Microbiol 29(10):2193–2196
37. Newcombe J, Cartwright K, Palmer WH et al. (1996) PCR of peripheral blood for diagnosis of meningococcal disease. J Clin Microbiol 34(7):1637–1640
38. Laforgia N, Coppola B, Carbone R et al. (1997) Rapid detection of neonatal sepsis using polymerase chain reaction. Acta Paediatr 86(10):1097–1099
39. Kempf VA, Trebesius K, Autenrieth IB (2000) Fluorescent In situ hybridization allows rapid identification of microorganisms in blood cultures. J Clin Microbiol 38(2):830–838
40. Jordan JA, Durso MB (2000) Comparison of 16S rRNA gene PCR and BACTEC 9240 for detection of neonatal bacteremia. J Clin Microbiol 38(7):2574–2578
41. Jansen GJ, Mooibroek M, Idema J et al. (2000) Rapid identification of bacteria in blood cultures by using fluorescently labeled oligonucleotide probes. J Clin Microbiol 38(2):814–817
42. Carroll KC, Leonard RB, Newcomb-Gayman PL et al. (1996) Rapid detection of the staphylococcal mecA gene from BACTEC blood culture bottles by the polymerase chain reaction. Am J Clin Pathol 106(5):600–605
43. Marlowe EM, Hogan JJ, Hindler JF et al. (2003) Application of an rRNA probe matrix for rapid identification of bacteria and fungi from routine blood cultures. J Clin Microbiol 41(11):5127–5133

44. Oliveira K, Haase G, Kurtzman C et al. (2001) Differentiation of Candida albicans and Candida dubliniensis by fluorescent in situ hybridization with peptide nucleic acid probes. J Clin Microbiol 39(11):4138–4141
45. Fredricks DN, Relman DA (1998) Improved amplification of microbial DNA from blood cultures by removal of the PCR inhibitor sodium polyanetholesulfonate. J Clin Microbiol 36(10):2810–2816
46. Moppett J, van dV, V, Wijkhuijs AJ et al. (2003) Inhibition affecting RQ-PCR-based assessment of minimal residual disease in acute lymphoblastic leukemia: reversal by addition of bovine serum albumin. Leukemia 17(1):268–270
47. Maes N, Magdalena J, Rottiers S et al. (2002) Evaluation of a triplex PCR assay to discriminate *Staphylococcus aureus* from coagulase-negative Staphylococci and determine methicillin resistance from blood cultures. J Clin Microbiol 40(4):1514–1517
48. Peters RP, van Agtmael MA, Danner SA et al. (2004) New developments in the diagnosis of bloodstream infections. Lancet Infect Dis 4(12):751–760
49. Cleven BE, Palka-Santini M, Gielen J et al. (2006) Identification and characterization of bacterial pathogens causing bloodstream infections by DNA microarray. J Clin Microbiol 44(7):2389–2397
50. Song JH, Cho H, Park MY et al. (1993) Detection of Salmonella typhi in the blood of patients with typhoid fever by polymerase chain reaction. J Clin Microbiol 31(6):1439–1443
51. Iralu JV, Sritharan VK, Pieciak WS et al. (1993) Diagnosis of *Mycobacterium avium* bacteremia by polymerase chain reaction. J Clin Microbiol 31(7):1811–1814
52. Wheeler J, Murphy OM, Freeman R et al. (2000) PCR can add to detection of pneumococcal disease in pneumonic patients receiving antibiotics at admission. J Clin Microbiol 38(10):3907
53. Lorente ML, Falguera M, Nogues A et al. (2000) Diagnosis of pneumococcal pneumonia by polymerase chain reaction (PCR) in whole blood: a prospective clinical study. Thorax 55(2):133–137
54. Zhang Y, Isaacman DJ, Wadowsky RM et al. (1995) Detection of *Streptococcus pneumoniae* in whole blood by PCR. J Clin Microbiol 33(3):596–601
55. Guiver M, Borrow R, Marsh J et al. (2000) Evaluation of the applied biosystems automated Taqman polymerase chain reaction system for the detection of meningococcal DNA. FEMS Immunol Med Microbiol 28(2):173–179
56. Schluger NW, Condos R, Lewis S et al. (1994) Amplification of DNA of *Mycobacterium tuberculosis* from peripheral blood of patients with pulmonary tuberculosis. Lancet 344(8917):232–233
57. Folgueira L, Delgado R, Palenque E et al. (1996) Rapid diagnosis of *Mycobacterium tuberculosis* bacteremia by PCR. J Clin Microbiol 34(3):512–515
58. Heininger A, Binder M, Schmidt S et al. (1999) PCR and blood culture for detection of *Escherichia coli* bacteremia in rats. J Clin Microbiol 37(8):2479–2482
59. van Burik JA, Myerson D, Schreckhise RW et al. (1998) Panfungal PCR assay for detection of fungal infection in human blood specimens. J Clin Microbiol 36(5):1169–1175
60. Wellinghausen N, Wirths B, Franz AR et al. (2004) Algorithm for the identification of bacterial pathogens in positive blood cultures by real-time LightCycler polymerase chain reaction (PCR) with sequence-specific probes. Diagn Microbiol Infect Dis 48(4):229–241
61. Klaschik S, Lehmann LE, Raadts A et al. (2004) Detection and differentiation of in vitro-spiked bacteria by real-time PCR and melting-curve analysis. J Clin Microbiol 42(2):512–517
62. Wisplinghoff H, Bischoff T, Tallent SM et al. (2004) Nosocomial bloodstream infections in US hospitals: analysis of 24,179 cases from a prospective nationwide surveillance study. Clin Infect Dis 39(3):309–317

63. Corless CE, Guiver M, Borrow R et al. (2001) Simultaneous detection of *Neisseria meningitidis, Haemophilus influenzae*, and *Streptococcus pneumoniae* in suspected cases of meningitis and septicemia using real-time PCR. J Clin Microbiol 39(4):1553–1558
64. Klaschik S, Lehmann LE, Raadts A et al. (2002) Real-time PCR for detection and differentiation of gram-positive and gram-negative bacteria. J Clin Microbiol 40(11):4304–4307
65. Lehmann LE, Hunfeld KP, Emrich T et al. (2008) A multiplex real-time PCR assay for rapid detection and differentiation of 25 bacterial and fungal pathogens from whole blood samples. Med Microbiol Immunol 197(3):313–324
66. Obaro SK, Madhi SA (2006) Bacterial pneumonia vaccines and childhood pneumonia: are we winning, refining, or redefining? Lancet Infect Dis 6(3):150–161
67. Rouphael NG, twell-Melnick N, Longo D et al. (2008) A real-time polymerase chain reaction for the detection of *Streptococcus pneumoniae* in blood using a mouse model: a potential new "gold standard". Diagn Microbiol Infect Dis 62(1):23–25
68. Hardie W, Bokulic R, Garcia VF et al. (1996) Pneumococcal pleural empyemas in children. Clin Infect Dis 22(6):1057–1063
69. Thomson AH, Hull J, Kumar MR et al. (2002) Randomised trial of intrapleural urokinase in the treatment of childhood empyema. Thorax 57(4):343–347
70. Salo P, Ortqvist A, Leinonen M (1995) Diagnosis of bacteremic pneumococcal pneumonia by amplification of pneumolysin gene fragment in serum. J Infect Dis 171(?):479–482
71. Tarrago D, Fenoll A, Sanchez-Tatay D et al. (2008) Identification of pneumococcal serotypes from culture-negative clinical specimens by novel real-time PCR. Clin Microbiol Infect 14(9):828–834
72. Harris KA, Turner P, Green EA et al. (2008) Duplex real-time PCR assay for detection of *Streptococcus pneumoniae* in clinical samples and determination of penicillin susceptibility. J Clin Microbiol 46(8):2751–2758
73. Corticelli AS, Di Nino GF, Gatti M et al. (1987) Intensive care units as a source of methicillin-resistant *Staphylococcus aureus*. Microbiologica 10(4):345–351
74. Guiguet M, Rekacewicz C, Leclercq B et al. (1990) Effectiveness of simple measures to control an outbreak of nosocomial methicillin-resistant *Staphylococcus aureus* infections in an intensive care unit. Infect Contr Hosp Epidemiol 11(1):23–26
75. Zhanel GG, DeCorby M, Laing N et al. (2008) Antimicrobial-resistant pathogens in intensive care units in Canada: results of the Canadian National Intensive Care Unit (CAN-ICU) study, 2005–2006. Antimicrob Agents Chemother 52(4):1430–1437
76. CDC – Centers for Disease Control and Prevention (1995) Recommendations for preventing spread of vancomycin resistance. Recommendations of the Hospital Infection Control Practices Advisory Committee (HICPAC). MMWR 44(RR12)1–13
77. Mayhall CG (1996) Prevention and control of vancomycin resistance in gram-positive coccal microorganisms: fire prevention and fire fighting. Infect Control Hosp Epidemiol 17(6):353–355
78. Stamper PD, Cai M, Howard T et al. (2007) Clinical validation of the molecular BD GeneOhm StaphSR assay for direct detection of *Staphylococcus aureus* and methicillin-resistant *Staphylococcus aureus* in positive blood cultures. J Clin Microbiol 45(7):2191–2196
79. Huletsky A, Giroux R, Rossbach V et al. (2004) New real-time PCR assay for rapid detection of methicillin-resistant *Staphylococcus aureus* directly from specimens containing a mixture of staphylococci. J Clin Microbiol 42(5):1875–1884
80. Thomas LC, Gidding HF, Ginn AN et al. (2007) Development of a real-time *Staphylococcus aureus* and MRSA (SAM-) PCR for routine blood culture. J Microbiol Methods 68(2):296–302
81. van Hal SJ, Jennings Z, Stark D et al. (2009) MRSA detection: comparison of two molecular methods (BD GeneOhm((R)) PCR assay and Easy-Plex) with two selective MRSA agars

(MRSA-ID and Oxoid MRSA) for nasal swabs. Eur J Clin Microbiol Infect Dis 28(1):47–53
82. Gurtler V, Stanisich VA (1996) New approaches to typing and identification of bacteria using the 16S-23S rDNA spacer region. Microbiology 142(Pt 1):3–16
83. Barry T, Glennon CM, Dunican LK et al. (1991) The 16s/23s ribosomal spacer region as a target for DNA probes to identify eubacteria. PCR Meth Appl 1(2):149
84. Kreger BE, Craven DE, Carling PC et al. (1980) Gram-negative bacteremia. III. Reassessment of etiology, epidemiology and ecology in 612 patients. Am J Med 68(3):332–343
85. Werner AS, Cobbs CG, Kaye D et al. (1967) Studies on the bacteremia of bacterial endocarditis. JAMA 202(3):199–203
86. Anderson BE, Sumner JW, Dawson JE et al. (1992) Detection of the etiologic agent of human ehrlichiosis by polymerase chain reaction. J Clin Microbiol 30(4):775–780
87. Arnoldi J, Schluter C, Duchrow M et al. (1992) Species-specific assessment of *Mycobacterium leprae* in skin biopsies by in situ hybridization and polymerase chain reaction. Lab Invest 66(5):618–623
88. Blanchard A, Gautier M, Mayau V (1991) Detection and identification of mycoplasmas by amplification of rDNA. FEMS Microbiol Lett 65(1):37–42
89. Boddinghaus B, Rogall T, Flohr T et al. (1990) Detection and identification of mycobacteria by amplification of rRNA. J Clin Microbiol 28(8):1751–1759
90. Kwok S, Higuchi R (1989) Avoiding false positives with PCR. Nature 339(6221):237–238
91. Bottger EC (1990) Frequent contamination of Taq polymerase with DNA. Clin Chem 36(6):1258–1259
92. Rand KH, Houck H (1990) Taq polymerase contains bacterial DNA of unknown origin. Mol Cell Probe 4(6):445–450
93. Schmidt TM, Pace B, Pace NR (1991) Detection of DNA contamination in Taq polymerase. Biotechniques 11(2):176–177
94. Meier A, Persing DH, Finken M et al. (1993) Elimination of contaminating DNA within polymerase chain reaction reagents: implications for a general approach to detection of uncultured pathogens. J Clin Microbiol 31(3):646–652
95. Jinno Y, Yoshiura K, Niikawa N (1990) Use of psoralen as extinguisher of contaminated DNA in PCR. Nucleic Acids Res 18(22):6739
96. Sarkar G, Sommer SS (1990) Shedding light on PCR contamination. Nature 343(6253):27
97. Ou CY, Moore JL, Schochetman G (1991) Use of UV irradiation to reduce false positivity in polymerase chain reaction. Biotechniques 10(4):442, 444, 446
98. Klaschik S, Lehmann LE, Raadts A et al. (2002) Comparison of different decontamination methods for reagents to detect low concentrations of bacterial 16S DNA by real-time-PCR. Mol Biotechnol 22(3):231–242
99. Vince A, Lepej SZ, Barsic B et al. (2008) LightCycler SeptiFast assay as a tool for the rapid diagnosis of sepsis in patients during antimicrobial therapy. J Med Microbiol 57(Pt 10):1306–1307
100. Mancini N, Clerici D, Diotti R et al. (2008) Molecular diagnosis of sepsis in neutropenic patients with haematological malignancies. J Med Microbiol 57(Pt 5):601–604
101. Mussap M, Molinari MP, Senno E et al. (2007) New diagnostic tools for neonatal sepsis: the role of a real-time polymerase chain reaction for the early detection and identification of bacterial and fungal species in blood samples. J Chemother 19(Suppl 2):31-4–31-34
102. Kane TD, Alexander JW, Johannigman JA (1998) The detection of microbial DNA in the blood: a sensitive method for diagnosing bacteremia and/or bacterial translocation in surgical patients. Ann Surg 227(1):1–9
103. Sleigh J, Cursons R, La PM (2001) Detection of bacteraemia in critically ill patients using 16S rDNA polymerase chain reaction and DNA sequencing. Intensive Care Med 27(8):1269–1273

104. Ley BE, Linton CJ, Bennett DM et al. (1998) Detection of bacteraemia in patients with fever and neutropenia using 16S rRNA gene amplification by polymerase chain reaction. Eur J Clin Microbiol Infect Dis 17(4):247–253
105. Cursons RT, Jeyerajah E, Sleigh JW (1999) The use of polymerase chain reaction to detect septicemia in critically ill patients. Crit Care Med 27(5):937–940
106. Corless CE, Guiver M, Borrow R et al. (2000) Contamination and sensitivity issues with a real-time universal 16S rRNA PCR. J Clin Microbiol 38(5):1747–1752
107. Berger SA, Weitzman S, Edberg SC et al. (1974) Bacteremia after the use of an oral irrigation device. A controlled study in subjects with normal-appearing gingiva: comparison with use of toothbrush. Ann Int Med 80(4):510–511
108. Bahrani-Mougeot FK, Paster BJ, Coleman S et al. (2008) Diverse and novel oral bacterial species in blood following dental procedures. J Clin Microbiol 46(6):2129–2132
109. Takeuchi T, Katsume A, Tanaka T et al. (1999) Real-time detection system for quantification of hepatitis C virus genome. Gastroenterology 116(3):636–642
110. Abe M, Klett C, Wieland E et al. (2008) Two-step real-time pcr quantification of all subtypes of human immunodeficiency virus type 1 by an in-house method using locked nucleic acid-based probes. Folia Med (Plovdiv) 50(3):5–13
111. Tedeschi R, Marus A, Bidoli E et al. (2008) Human herpesvirus 8 DNA quantification in matched plasma and PBMCs samples of patients with HHV8-related lymphoproliferative diseases. J Clin Virol 43(3):255–259
112. Malnati MS, Scarlatti G, Gatto F et al. (2008) A universal real-time PCR assay for the quantification of group-M HIV-1 proviral load. Nat Protoc 3(7):1240–1248
113. Hackett SJ, Carrol ED, Guiver M et al. (2002) Improved case confirmation in meningococcal disease with whole blood Taqman PCR. Arch Dis Child 86(6):449–452
114. Hackett SJ, Guiver M, Marsh J et al. (2002) Meningococcal bacterial DNA load at presentation correlates with disease severity. Arch Dis Child 86(1):44–46

Influence of Serotype in Pneumococcal Disease: A New Challenge for Vaccination

Manel Luján, Yolanda Belmonte, and Dionisia Fontanals

1
Introduction

Streptococcus pneumoniae is one of the most important causes of morbidity and mortality worldwide. It is responsible for the severe infectious clinical pictures seen in, for example, bacteremic pneumonia (BPP), meningitis, and bacteremia of unknown source.

The polysaccharide capsule, which protects the microorganism against phagocytosis, is considered to be the primary virulence factor of pneumococci, because although pneumococcus exists is encapsulated and unencapsulated forms, only encapsulated strains have been recovered from clinical specimens. Classic studies carried out by Avery [1] demonstrated that loss of the capsule is accompanied by a 100,000-fold reduction in the virulence of the pneumococci. On the basis of differences in capsular polysaccharide structure, pneumococci can be divided into more than 90 serotypes, but fewer than 30 serotypes account for up to 90% of invasive diseases in humans [2].

For many years, the main efforts in studies on pneumococcal disease have been directed toward antibiotic therapy for infected patients, but they have not significantly reduced the burden of infection, and, in the last two decades, interest has also been focused on preventive strategies against pneumococcal disease.

The active immunization against *S. pneumoniae* is currently founded on two approaches, both based on purified extracts of the pneumococcal capsule, the same structure that classifies pneumococci into different serotypes: the capsular polysaccharide pneumococcal vaccines (PPV) and the conjugate pneumococcal vaccines (PCV).

M. Luján (✉)
Department of Pneumology, Hospital de Sabadell, Parc Taulí, s/n. 08208 – Sabadell, Spain
e-mail: mlujan@tauli.cat

2
Current Situation of Active Immunization Against *S. pneumoniae*: An Overview

2.1
The Pneumococcal Polysaccharide Vaccine PPV-23

The PPV-23 vaccine was licensed in 1983, and contains capsular polysaccharide antigens from the 23 most prevalent serotypes (Table 1) of *S. pneumoniae* in clinical isolates, encompassing about 90% of isolated types in invasive pneumococcal disease (IPD). After administration, it induces type-specific antibodies, through a T-cell-independent mechanism, which enhances opsonization and phagocytosis. Currently, the administration of PPV-23 is recommended in elderly subjects (older than 65 years) or younger patients with comorbidities [3]. However, several points remain unclear about the immunological properties and the efficacy of the PPV-23 vaccine. Some of the concerns regarding the immunological response of vaccinated subjects include:

- The immunological quantitative response is heterogeneous among different serotypes included in the vaccine. For example, titers against serotypes 7, 14, and 19 F are higher than those against serotypes 1 or 4. These findings support the concept that PPV-23 is in fact 23 different vaccines in a single dose [4].
- The response is also heterogeneous between different subjects. Immunocompromised patients, very elderly subjects (older than 80 years), and probably chronic obstructive pulmonary disease patients are poor responders to PPV-23 [5, 6].
- The level of antibodies that provide protection against infection is unknown. Moreover, the determination of functional levels is technically difficult, because most elderly people have acquired nonfunctional antibodies [7].

Table 1 Current licensed vaccines, vaccines under development, and serotypes included in each formulation

Currently licensed							
23 Valent polysaccharide (PPV-23)	1	2	3	4	5	6B	
	7F	8	9N	9V	10A	11A	
	12F	14	15B	17F	18C	19F	
	19A	20	22F	23F	33F		
7 Valent conjugated	4	6B	9V	14	18C	19F	
	23F						
Not licensed							
9 Valent conjugated	1	4	5	6B	9V	14	
	18C	19F	23F				
10 Valent conjugated	1	4	5	6B	7F		
	9V	14	18C	19F	23F		
13 Valent conjugated	1	3	4	5	6A	6B	7F
	9V	14	18C	19A	19F	23F	

However, the limitations of PPV-23 are not only related to its immunological behavior, but also to the protective effects of the administration. Thus, although it has been demonstrated [8] that PPV-23 provides protection against invasive pneumococcal disease – the meta-analysis of Dear and coworkers [9] showed a protection of more than 50% for a cohort of patients aged over 65 – the effectiveness in protection against nonbacteremic infections is still unclear. The difficulty of verifying the pneumococcal etiology in patients with nonbacteremic pneumonia is the main drawback in evaluating the effect of PPV-23. For this reason, and assuming that a great number of patients with pneumonia of unknown etiology have in fact pneumococcal pneumonia, most studies have evaluated the effect of PPV-23 in overall pneumonia. Only one of them [10] has demonstrated a reduction in the risk of hospitalization and death from pneumonia and a protective effect against nonbacteremic pneumococcal pneumonia (39% of reduction).

Another controversial topic is the need and time for revaccination. It is well known that the effectiveness provided by PPV-23 against pneumococcal bacteremia declines over time [6], and revaccination is recommended [3] after an interval of 5 years or less. However, the level of specific antibodies after revaccination seems significantly lower than that achieved after the first vaccination [4], and there is concern that, although revaccination leads to a moderate increase of antibody levels, the administration of a first dose of unconjugated vaccine may blunt the immune response to second or third doses. This effect is also seen in patients receiving a single dose of conjugated vaccine (PCV-7) after administration of a previous unconjugated PPV-23 vaccine [11]. It remains to be demonstrated whether this phenomenon correlates with lower protection, although early studies in a revaccinated population [12, 13] did not find any reduction in the protective effects of PPV-23 after a revaccination.

2.2
The Pneumococcal Conjugated Vaccine PCV-7

The PPV-23 vaccine showed poor immunogenicity after administration in young children. The conjugate pneumococcal vaccines, in which polysaccharides are bound to protein carriers, have been shown to be immunogenic and preventive of pneumococcal disease in children. In 2000, a conjugate vaccine including the most prevalent serotypes in the pediatric population (Table 1) was licensed for use in children.

Studies in the pediatric population after the licensing of PCV-7 demonstrated an important reduction in invasive disease. Whitney and coworkers reported an effectiveness of 96% against vaccine serotypes in healthy children and 81% in those with underlying comorbidities [14]. Even in immunosuppressed patients, the vaccine provided 65% protection against serotypes included in the vaccine [15].

The PCV-7 vaccine also prevents the asymptomatic carriage of pneumococcus in the nasopharynx. Children are the main reservoir for pneumococci, and probably represent the source of spread to adults, especially to the elderly. Thus, the above-mentioned effects after licensure of PCV-7 were also noted in the nonvaccinated adult population (herd immunity effect). Whitney and coworkers found a significant reduction in the prevalence of invasive pneumococcal disease in adults after PCV-7 licensure, with this reduction being especially important in the cohort of elderly people [16]. Similarly, Hicks and coworkers [17] reported a significant reduction in IPD after PCV was licensed (from 61 cases of IPD/100,000 population in 1999 to 38/100,000 in 2004). This effect was mainly due to a great reduction of IPD caused by PCV-7 serotypes (34.5 cases/100,000 in 1999 to 8,2 in 2004). In this study, the absolute number of IPD cases caused by non-PCV-7 serotypes increased only slightly.

When the PCV-7 vaccine was administered directly to an adult population, in pneumococcal vaccine-naive adults aged over 70, de Roux and coworkers [11] found higher ELISA geometric mean concentrations and opsonophagocytic activity for the seven serotypes common to PCV-7 and PPV-23 when compared with patients that received PPV-23. This immunological response seems to be dose-dependent, especially in adults previously vaccinated with PPV-23. Jackson et al. found an increase in antibody response in elderly individuals who received twice the standard dose of PCV-7 [18].

Finally, and due to the low number of serotypes included in the PCV-7 vaccine, the geographic distribution of serotypes is a key point for predicting the effectiveness of the vaccine. In the United States the PCV7 serotypes accounted for more than 90% of IPD among children, whereas in Western Europe it was only 18–43% [19].

2.3
The "Replacement Phenomenon" After PCV-7 Administration

In recent years, a serotype replacement phenomenon has been observed, in which decreases in disease caused by vaccine-type serotypes are counterbalanced by increases in disease due to nonvaccine serotypes. This phenomenon seems to be independent of the geographic area studied. Thus, Singleton and coworkers [13, 20] studied the distribution of serotypes in native Alaskan children after PCV-7 vaccination. The prevalence of nasopharyngeal colonization remained stable over time (around 40% in periods before and after PCV-7 administration) but, while in the PCV serotypes a significant reduction was found (41–5%), it was counterbalanced by an increase in non-PCV-7 types (47–88%). For example, the prevalence of children colonized by serotype 19A (not included in PCV-7) increased from 0.5% of cases in 1998 to 15% in 2004. In the same study, these findings were also observed in IPD.

In Europe, a recent study [21] demonstrated that in the years preceding the licensure of PCV-7, the PCV serotypes accounted for 39.9% of IPD. This percentage remained stable in the early PCV-7 period (33.6%), but decreased in the late PCV-7 period (21%, $p < 0.001$). In contrast, rates of IPD due to seven non-PCV serotypes significantly increased (serotypes 1, 5, 7F, 12 F, 19 A, 22 F, and 24). This study also confirms that the increase in the incidence of IPD due to non-PCV-7 serotypes is related to dissemination of specific clones of these non-PCV-7 serotypes. Finally, another important finding in this study was the decrease in the proportion of antibiotic-resistant pneumococci after introduction of PCV-7, because of the high prevalence of antimicrobial resistance of the PCV-7 serotypes. Of note, Kiaw and colleagues reported the same finding in the United States [22] among persons of 65 years of age or older. These authors found a 49% decline in the disease (16.4–8.4 cases per 100,000) caused by penicillin nonsusceptible strains.

Thus, the replacement of serotypes following the introduction of universal vaccination of children with PCV-7 represents an important change in the ecology of pneumococcal disease. And the consequences are not the simple replacement of some serotypes for others. Several authors have reported specific clinical issues linked to this replacement. For example, Bender and coworkers reported an increasing number of children with necrotizing pneumonia caused by serotype 3 [23], an increasing number of cases of pleural empyema have been also reported associated to serotype 1, and mastoiditis and recalcitrant acute otitis media due to multidrug-resistant serotype 19A has also been noted [24].

3
Serotypes of *Streptococcus pneumoniae*: Are They Clinically Different?

Individual serotypes seem to have not only geographic differences, but also differences in the potential to cause invasive disease (invasiveness) and probably severe disease (virulence). In an early adult case series, unadjusted mortality rates from invasive disease were increased in patients infected by certain serotypes. In the study of Austrian and Gold [25], the authors correlated the serotype, age, presence of preexisting illness, and pulmonary consolidation with mortality in bacteremic pneumococcal pneumonia. The fatality rate for serotype 1 was 8%, whereas it was 55% for serotype 3 infection. The rate of mortality due to infection with other serotypes was in the range of 15–25%. Even when adjustments were made for age, the mortality after infection with pneumococcus type 3 was severalfold higher than that for infection with any other serotype. Among patients infected with serotype 3, the mortality was concentrated in older patients with comorbidities, and these patients did not show an increased prevalence of infection by any concrete serotype.

Three decades later, Henriques et al. [26] conducted a multicenter international study, involving five healthcare centers in five different countries. An increased case-fatality rate for serotypes 3, 6B, and 19F (25%) was found in this study, but the mortality was not adjusted for other potential confounding factors, mainly age or comorbidity. Other serotypes, such as 1 and 7F, presented a lower mortality (0% of case-fatality rate). After controlling for other factors related to outcome, Martens and coworkers [27] studied retrospectively 464 patients with pneumococcal invasive disease, and found that serotype 3 was linked to higher mortality in the global cohort (OR = 2.63), but only a trend ($p = 0.06$) was seen in patients with pneumonia. The cohort of patients with pneumonia presented a very high mortality (27%), but, surprisingly, only 10% received mechanical ventilation, perhaps indicating a therapeutic limitation that can influence outcome.

In contrast, more recently, Alanee et al. [28] in an international study including 796 patients did not find any association between mortality and specific serotypes, indicating that in their study, host factors were more important than strain in determining the severity and outcome. Severity was assessed by means of the Pitt bacteremia score, and only preexisting lung disease, meningitis, and suppurative complications were independent risk factors for a Pitt bacteremia score of more than 4; independent risk factors for mortality were older age, underlying comorbidity, immunosuppression, and severity of illness at admission. The groups of capsular types were classified as follows: pediatric serotypes (6, 9, 14, 19, and 23), conjugate serotypes (those included in PCV-7), and invasive serotypes (1, 5 and 7F).

All these studies were focused mainly on the influence of infecting serotypes on outcome. Related to invasiveness, epidemiological studies comparing the distribution of invasive isolates with carriage isolates have also shown that the potential for pneumococci to cause invasive disease differs by serotype. In the meta-analysis conducted by Brueggemann [29], the odds ratio (OR) for causing invasive disease (in a pediatric population) for different serotypes was investigated. Certain serotypes, such as 1 and 7F, were frequently associated with invasive disease, but were rarely associated with colonization of the nasopharynx. Other serotypes, such as 3, 6A, 6B, 8, 19F, and 23F, are more commonly carried in the nasopharynx, but rarely caused invasive disease. Of note, three of these serotypes are those that were associated with higher mortality in the study by Henriques (3, 6B, and 19 F). In a recent editorial, Garau and Calbo [30] suggested that the higher invasive disease potential of some serotypes (1 and 7F) might be secondary to the lack of a pilus-like structure in their capsule. Briefly, pili structures project from the bacterial cell surface, and are found in some – but not all – pneumococcal strains. Pili expression also augments the host's inflammatory response. Thus, strains that lack pili (i.e., strains that belong to clones of serotypes 1 and 7F) may cause invasive disease of a relatively mild character. In contrast, pili-positive pneumococcal strains of type 4 and 19F are associated with a high cytokine response, probably increasing the severity of the infected patients.

But is there a relationship between invasiveness and outcome? In a recent study, Sjostrom et al. [31] reported that the different serotypes not only had a different case-fatality rate, but disease severity and disease type were also different according to the infecting serotype Checked and confirmed. Moreover, other factors, such as age and the presence of underlying comorbidity, influenced the isolation of one or another serotype. Thus, serotype 1 was isolated mainly in young people, whereas serotype 23F infected older patients (>65 years old). Certain serotypes (11A, 19 A, 6A) infected mainly patients with comorbidity, whereas others (mainly serotype 1) infected previously healthy people.

When the serotypes were grouped according to the invasiveness criteria proposed by Brueggemann, it was concluded that there were serotypes that acted as "primary pathogens" infecting previously healthy people (those with "high invasive disease potential", mainly 1 and 7F) but caused paradoxically milder disease, whereas other serotypes acted as "opportunistic pathogens," infecting patients with comorbidity and being associated with an increased case-fatality rate.

In our experience in the last 9 years with a model of bacteremic pneumococcal pneumonia, we also found significant differences in the clinical behavior of several serotypes of pneumococci. The infecting serotype was determined in 243 of 248 patients. Figure 1 shows the distribution of the serotypes: serotypes 1, 3, and 14 were the most prevalent in the cohort. Our purpose was to clarify whether the isolation of certain serotypes was associated with increased 30-day mortality. The main findings are summarized as follows:

Firstly, using the 2008 CLSI breakpoints, nonsusceptibility to penicillin (MIC ≥ 4 mg ml^{-1}) was documented in only 3 of 248 (1.5%) episodes. Three isolates were also documented as being resistant to cephalosporins. Resistance to macrolides was 18%. As a consequence of this low percentage of resistances, only two patients received inappropriate empirical therapy.

Then, the infecting serotypes were grouped according to the invasiveness criteria proposed by Brueggemann and coworkers in their meta-analysis. Patients infected with

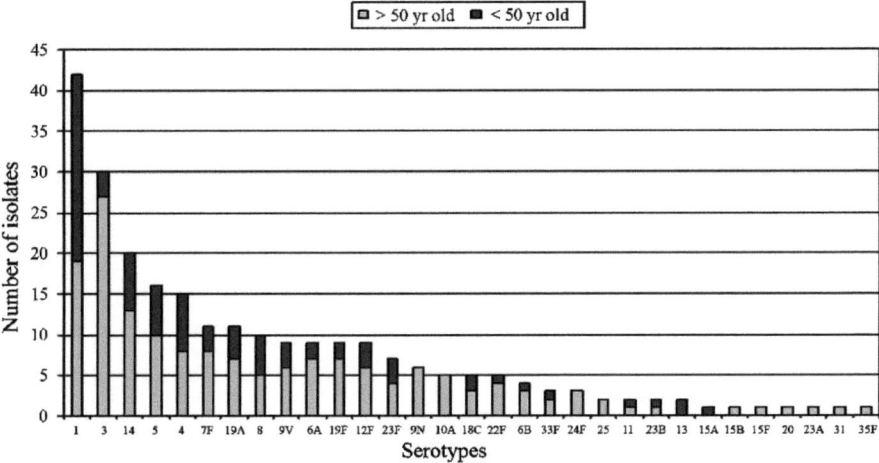

Fig. 1 Distribution of serotypes in the overall cohort and between different age-groups in a study including 248 patients with bacteremic pneumococcal pneumonia

"high invasive disease potential" (1, 5, 7F) were younger, previously healthy, and presented lower severity and mortality, but had a significantly higher incidence of empyema (16% vs. 3%). Moreover, in a multivariate model, only infection by invasive serotypes reached statistical significance as an independent risk factor for developing empyema (OR = 4.36 95% CI 1.32–14.42).

Conversely, the patients infected with serotypes associated with "low invasive disease potential" (3, 6A, 6B, 8, 19F, and 23F) did not exhibit the same clinical signs as those infected with serotypes 1, 5, and 7F. In contrast to previous studies, patients infected with these serotypes were not significantly older and did not have more comorbidities; however, they presented with not only higher mortality, but also more frequently with severe pneumonia (PSI V), were more likely to have a PaO_2/FiO_2 ratio below 250 at admission, and had a greater need for mechanical ventilation, vasopressors, and ICU admission. Of interest, the subset of patients with comorbidities infected with these serotypes also had a higher mortality than patients with comorbidities infected with other serotypes (35.2% vs. 9% OR = 5.25 95% CI 2.25–12.24), and the number of comorbidities was not different in both groups (1.5 vs. 1.47 p = ns). When the infection by these serotypes was adjusted for underlying disease and severity-of-illness at admission in a Cox proportional hazard model, it remained an independent factor of mortality (see Table 2). Thus, the infection by serotypes classified as having "low invasive disease potential" increased the probability of death 2.5-fold.

At the same time, we analyzed the potential impact of vaccination with the conjugated vaccines, the licensed PCV-7 and the newer PCV-13, currently being included in a pilot clinical trial for people aged 50 or more. When we analyzed the entire cohort, neither the PCV-7 nor the PCV-13 serotypes were associated with increased 30-day mortality. These results were in agreement with those reported by Alanee [28]. However, when we analyzed the cohort of patients aged 50 years or more, both groups of serotypes (7 and 13) were associated with increased 30-day mortality. Finally, when the model was adjusted for the

Table 2 Cox proportional hazard ratio for mortality (censored at 30 days) in a study including 248 patients with bacteremic pneumococcal pneumonia

Variables	OR for death	CI 95%	p value
Prior hospitalization	4.51	2.04–9.95	< 0.001
$PaO_2/FiO_2 < 250$	3.51	1.13–8.51	< 0.05
Infection by serotypes having low invasive disease potential	2.54	1.18–5.46	0.01

Serotypes classified as having low invasive disease potential were 3, 6A, 6B, 8, 19 F, and 23 F, in accordance with Brueggemann and coworkers [29]

covariables (underlying condition and severity-of-illness) related with mortality in the univariate model, both capsular groups remained independently associated with mortality. Moreover, if we assume a 100% efficacy of PCV-13 in the cohort of adults aged over 50 years, then administration of this vaccine may prevent up to 80% of deaths in this subgroup.

In summary, the analyzed studies suggest that capsular types of pneumococci may have important differences in their association with mortality. To date, the prevention of pneumococcal disease has been based on strictly epidemiological criteria. It is probably time to take into account the data on severity and mortality provided by these studies, especially in the elderly population. The new PCV-13 vaccine may cover three key points in the prevention of pneumococcal disease in adults: first, it has been demonstrated to be more immunogenic, even in poor-responders to PPV-23; second, its formulation includes the vast majority of serotypes associated with increased mortality in the elderly; and third, it may fight against the new and severe clinical pictures caused by the spread of clonal types not included in PCV-7. However, there is a reasonable doubt over its introduction in daily practice: should we administer the vaccine to adults, seeking a direct immunogenic effect, or might eradication in the pediatric population be enough through the herd immunity effect?

4
Conclusions

1. The nonconjugated vaccines provide suboptimal immunologic protection in elderlyWW people and in the immunocompromised host. Moreover, although it protects against invasive pneumococcal disease, it provides less protection against nonbacteremic pneumococcal pneumonia.
2. The conjugated vaccines are more immunogenic in children and probably in previously nonvaccinated adults. After PCV-7 licensure and administration in children, the prevalence of colonization and pneumococcal infection by the serotypes included in this vaccine in the pediatric population has decreased dramatically. Moreover, through the herd immunity effect, the prevalence of IPD in adults caused by PCV serotypes has also decreased in the last 4 years. Moreover, since the PCV-7 serotypes are associated with nonsusceptibility to antibiotics, the administration of PCV-7 may be one of the causes of the reduction in resistance reported in recent studies.

3. The replacement phenomenon is not only a change of some serotypes by others. The clonal expansion of non-PCV-7 serotypes results in newer and sometimes severe clinical pictures. The epidemiological surveillance of the replacement phenomenon should provide important information for the design and licensure of new vaccines.
4. The design of conjugated vaccines is based on epidemiological criteria in the pediatric population. If we consider the administration of conjugated vaccines to adults, the influence of the serotypes on outcome should be considered.

References

1. Avery OT, Dubos R. The protective action of a specific enzyme against type III pneumococcus infection in mice. J Exp Med 1931: 54:73–89
2. Henrichsen J. Six newly recognized types of *Streptococcus pneumoniae*. J Clin Microbiol 1995; 33:2759–2762
3. Mandell LA, Wunderink RG, Anzueto A, et al. Infectious Diseases Society of America; American Thoracic Society. Infectious Diseases Society of America/American Thoracic Society consensus guidelines on the management of community-acquired pneumonia in adults. Clin Infect Dis 2007; 44:S27–S72
4. Torling J, Hedlund J, Konradsen HB, Ortqvist A. Revaccination with the 23-valent pneumococcal polysaccharide vaccine in middle-aged and elderly persons previously treated for pneumonia. Vaccine 2003; 22:96–103
5. Schenkein JG, Nahm MH, Dransfield MT. Pneumococcal vaccination for patients with COPD: current practice and future directions. Chest 2008; 133:767–774
6. Shapiro ED, Berg AT, Austrian R, et al. The protective efficacy of polyvalent pneumococcal polysaccharide vaccine. N Engl J Med 1991; 325:1453–1460
7. Coughlin RT, White AC, Anderson CA, et al. Characterization of pneumococcal specific antibodies in healthy unvaccinated adults. Vaccine 1998; 16:1761–1767
8. Jackson LA, Neuzil KM, Yu O, et al. Effectiveness of pneumococcal polysaccharide vaccine in older adults. N Engl J Med 2003; 348:1747–1755
9. Dear K, Holden J, Andrews R, Tatham D. Vaccines for preventing pneumococcal infection in adults. Cochrane Database Syst Rev 2003 (4) CD000422
10. Vila-Corcoles A, Ochoa-Gondar O, Hospital I, et al. Protective effects of the 23-valent pneumococcal polysaccharide vaccine in the elderly population: the EVAN-65 study. Clin Infect Dis 2006; 43:860–868
11. de Roux A, Schmoele-Thoma B, Siber GR, et al. Comparison of pneumococcal conjugate polysaccharide and free polysaccharide vaccines in elderly adults: conjugate vaccine elicits improved antibacterial immune responses and immunological memory. Clin Infect Dis 2008; 46:1015–1023
12. Benin AL, O'Brien KL, Watt JP, et al. Effectiveness of the 23-valent polysaccharide vaccine against invasive pneumococcal disease in Navajo adults. J Infect Dis 2003; 188:81–89
13. Singleton RJ, Butler JC, Bulkow LR, et al. Invasive pneumococcal disease epidemiology and effectiveness of 23-valent pneumococcal polysaccharide vaccine in Alaska native adults. Vaccine 2007; 25:2288–2295
14. Whitney CG, Pilishvili T Farley MM, et al. Efectiveness of seven valent pneumococcal conjugated vaccine against invasive pneumococcal disease: a matched case-control study. Lancet 2006: 368:1495–1502
15. Klugman KP, Madhi SA, Huebner RE, et al. A trial of a 9-valent pneumococcal conjugate vaccine in children with and those without HIV infection. N Engl J Med 2003; 349: 1341–1348

16. Whitney CG, Farley MM, Hadler J, et al. Decline in invasive pneumococcal disease after the introduction of protein-polysaccharide conjugate vaccine. N Engl J Med 2003; 348:1737–1746
17. Hicks LA, Harrison LH, Flannery B, et al. Incidence of pneumococcal disease due to non-pneumococcal conjugate vaccine (PCV7) serotypes in the United States during the era of widespread PCV7 vaccination, 1998–2004. J Infect Dis 2007; 196:1346–1354
18. Jackson LA, Neuzil KM, Nahm MH, et al. Immunogenicity of varying dosages of 7-valent pneumococcal polysaccharide-protein conjugate vaccine in seniors previously vaccinated with 23-valent pneumococcal polysaccharide vaccine. Vaccine 2007; 25:4029–4037
19. Jefferson T, Ferroni E, Curtale F, et al. *Streptococcus pneumoniae* in western Europe: serotype distribution and incidence in children less than 2 years old. Lancet Infect Dis 2006, 6:405–410
20. Singleton RJ, Hennessy TW, Bulkow LR, et al. Invasive pneumococcal disease caused by nonvaccine serotypes among Alaska native children with high levels of 7-valent pneumococcal conjugate vaccine coverage. JAMA 2007; 297:1784–1792
21. Ardanuy C, Tubau F, Pallarés R, et al. Epidemiology of invasive pneumococcal disease among adult patients in Barcelona before and after pediatric 7-valent pneumococcal conjugate vaccine introduction, 1997–2007. CID 2009; 48:57–64
22. Kyaw MH, Lynfield R, Schaffner W, et al. Effect of introduction of the pneumococcal conjugate vaccine on drug-resistant *Streptococcus pneumoniae*. N Engl J Med 2006; 354:1455–1463
23. Bender JM, Ampofo K, Korgenski K. Pneumococcal necrotizing pneumonia in Utah: does serotype matter? Clin Infect Dis 2008: 46: 1346–1352
24. Pichichero ME, Casey JR. Emergence of a multiresistant serotype 19 A pneumococcal strain not included in the 7-valent conjugate vaccine as an otopathogen in children. JAMA 2007; 298:1772–1778
25. Austrian R, Gold J. Pneumococcal bacteremia with special reference to bacteremic pneumococcal pneumonia. Ann Int Med 1964; 60:759–776
26. Henriques B, Kalin M, Ortqvist A, et al. Molecular epidemiology of *Streptococcus pneumoniae* causing invasive disease in 5 countries. J Infect Dis 2000; 182:833–839
27. Martens P, Worm SW, Lundgren B, et al. Serotype-specific mortality from invasive *Streptococcus pneumoniae* disease revisited. BMC Infect Dis 2004; 30(4):21–28
28. Alanee SR, McGee L, Jackson D, et al. Association of serotypes of *Streptococcus pneumoniae* with disease severity and outcome in adults: an international study. Clin Infect Dis 2007; 45:46–51
29. Brueggemann AB, Griffiths DT, Meats E, et al. Clonal relationships between invasive and carriage *Streptococcus pneumoniae* and serotype and clone-specific differences in invasive potential. J Infect Dis 2003 187:1424–1432
30. Garau J, Calbo E. Capsular types and predicting patient outcomes in pneumococcal bacteremia. Clin Infect Dis 2007, 45:52–54
31. Sjöström K, Spindler C, Ortqvist A, et al. Clonal and capsular types decide whether pneumococci will act as a primary or opportunistic pathogen. Clin Infect Dis 2006; 42:451–459

Acute Kidney Injury and Extracorporeal Blood Purification in Sepsis

8

Javier Maynar Moliner, José Ángel Sánchez-Izquierdo Riera, Manuel Herrera Gutiérrez, Amaia Quintano Rodero, and Alberto Manzano Ramirez

1 Introduction

Acute renal failure (ARF) occurs when the kidneys fail to eliminate nitrogenous waste products and to maintain homeostasis of water and electrolytes [1]. The consequences of this derangement can (if not reversed on time) precipitate a syndrome that can interfere with the already difficult management of intensive care unit (ICU) septic patients and worsen their prognosis.

Historically, many different definitions have been provided for ARF in different studies, which makes it difficult to compare experiences and explains the wide range of figures reported on incidence or mortality. The concept is still evolving, but recently some consensus has been reached that allows us to define our understanding of ARF, or even better of acute kidney injury (AKI). The term "acute kidney injury" is a step forward that stresses the necessity to detect and provide support for this problem in the early stages of the process, before there is complete failure of the kidneys.

As stated, the main problem in addressing the epidemiology of AKI is the lack of consensus on the definition of this process [2]. It is universally accepted that uncomplicated AKI as a whole is a process with a low incidence and a good prognosis. Although this statement is generally true (the mortality rate is under 5%) [3], we must accept that AKI is not an accompanying phenomenon and that per se it affects survival independently and significantly. In a recent study by Levy et al. on patients undergoing procedures with radiocontrast agents, the investigators detected that ARF was associated with an odds ratio of 5.5 for mortality [4]. Moreover, when AKI develops in the hospital setting it is associated with poorer outcome [5], and in these cases, hypovolemia, ischemia, or toxic acute tubular necrosis (ATN) is the predominant cause [6].

J.M. Moliner (✉)
Department of Intensive Care Medicine, Santiago Apóstol Hospital, Vitoria, Spain,
franciscojavier.maynarmoliner@osakidetza.net

The prevalence of ARF in ICUs approaches 5% in most studies (5.7% in the multicenter international study BEST or 5.6% in Spanish ICUs), and when septic shock is present, prevalence is over 50% [6–8]. Mortality is over 40% and higher than that predicted by SAPS II, and when complicated by severe sepsis in the ICU mortality rises to 50–70%. These figures have not improved for several decades [5, 9]. On the other hand, more than 85% of patients who survive the episode are dialysis-independent at discharge.

2
AKI and Sepsis

The exact mechanisms and sequence of events resulting in renal dysfunction in sepsis are poorly understood, but we know that over 90% of AKI episodes in the ICU are either prerenal dysfunction or ATN [6] and these two processes share a common origin: hypoperfusion. Sepsis induces cytokine-mediated (tumor necrosis factor, interleukin-1, and chemokines) nitric oxide synthesis leading to a decrease in systemic vascular resistance. This implies a low effective circulating volume, predisposing patients to acute renal failure. This environment could be worsened by loss of fluids (third space, hemorrhage, etc.) and/or low cardiac performance. In addition, this arterial vasodilatation is sometimes resistant to exogenous catecholamine. An increase of hydrogen ions and lactate in plasma concentrations and a decrease of ATP in vascular smooth muscle cells cause hyperpolarization of the vascular smooth muscle cells. Furthermore, the high endogenous levels of vasoactive hormones during sepsis may be associated with downregulation of their receptors, which would result in a weakening of their effects on the vasculature. Furthermore angiotensin II and endothelin, which try to support arterial tone, also cause renal vasoconstriction and predispose patients to acute renal failure [10]. The procoagulant state seen in sepsis can also lead to disseminated intravascular coagulation, which is related to glomerular thrombi and acute renal failure.

Regarding the clinical impact of this relationship, sepsis is the main predisposing factor for AKI development in the ICU [11], and AKI is present in more than 50% of patients with septic shock [12]; this figure could be even higher if we look closely for its presence [13]. As already stated, the combination of AKI and sepsis is associated with up to 70% mortality, as compared with 45% mortality among patients with AKI alone. Finally, it is also recognized that untreated ARF may contribute to a higher incidence of new-onset sepsis [4].

3
Definition and Stratification of AKI

It can be said that there are as many definitions of AKI as studies published. Moreover, until recently all the diagnostic criteria were based on isolated determinations of different markers for renal function with arbitrary levels for defining abnormality.

A sensible definition for AKI could be: "a sudden loss of renal function followed by alterations in electrolyte, acid–base, and fluid homeostasis". This seems a clear statement but is prone to different interpretations: What do we understand by "sudden"? Which parameters can be applied for better measurement of the decline? Should we considerer urine flow in the diagnosis? [14].

The Acute Dialysis Quality Initiative (ADQI) Group proposed a new definition of AKI [15] as a "sudden and maintained decline in glomerular filtration rate (GFR), urine flow or both," and addressed all these questions with a novel approach that takes into account the following: we must consider changes from baseline status; the system must be easy to use and must consider acute on chronic failure; and, finally, should allow detection of patients in whom renal function is mildly affected and patients in whom renal function is markedly affected.

Based on these premises, a multilevel classification system was proposed that fulfills these criteria and in which a wide range of disease spectra can be included: the multilevel classification RIFLE (Table 1). The RIFLE classification seems to be an adequate tool for monitoring changes in renal injury and (according to some studies) as a marker for prognosis as well. In a study by Hoste et al., patients with RIFLE class R had a mortality rate of 8.8%, class I 11.4%, and class F 26.3%, compared with 5.5% without AKI. Those cases with RIFLE R were at high risk of progression to class I or class F (more than 50% progressed to a higher level) [13]. In a retrospective study of 15,019 patients, those with R had hospital mortality rates of 20.9%, with I 45.6%, and with F 56.8% compared with 8.4% among patients without AKI [16]. All these studies were based only on changes in serum creatinine (Cr_s) level; it is not possible to say whether the inclusion of urine output criteria could show different results, but some data point to the possibility that the RIFLE score based on GFR criteria predicts a slightly higher hospital mortality than when based on urine output (27.9% vs. 21.9%) [13].

These studies used the RIFLE system based on the worst measure during the stay. As an earlier marker, RIFLE has been studied by Ahlstrom et al. during the first 3 ICU days, and they found that hospital mortality increased from 13% in the R group to 23% in patients with F. In our experience, the RIFLE system based on Cr_s during the first 24 h of ICU stay was not reliable as a marker for mortality, but when calculated using creatinine clearance (CrCl) instead of Cr_s it showed a good correlation with mortality (as an expression of the delay in the rise of Cr_s after the decline of GFR) [17].

Table 1 RIFLE classification [15]

Group	Glomerular filtration rate criteria	Urine output criteria
Risk	↑ Cr_s × 1.5 or ↑ CrCl > 25%	<0.5 mL kg^{-1} h^{-1} × 6 h
Injury	↑ Cr_s × 2 or ↑ CrCl > 50%	<0.5 mL kg^{-1} h^{-1} × 12 h <0.3 mL kg^{-1} h^{-1} × 24 h or anuria × 12 h
Failure	↑ Cr_s × 3 or ↑ CrCl > 75% or Cr_s ≥ 4 mgr dL^{-1}	
Loss	Persistent ARF = loss > 4 weeks	
Eskd	>3 months	

GRF glomerular filtration rate; *Cr_s* serum creatinine; *Eskd* end-stage kidney disease; *ARF* acute renal failure

Emerging evidence suggests that changes in Cr_s as low as 0.3–0.4 mg dL^{-1} are associated with increased in-hospital mortality [18, 19]. This fact and the need for earlier detection of the renal derangement have led to the redefinition of the RIFLE criteria to include a 48-h window for the first documentation of the increase in Cr_s and to include increments of more than 0.3 mg dL^{-1}: the Acute Kidney Injury Network (AKIN) classification (Table 2) [20].

SIRO, an interesting approach which is similar to that proposed in the PIRO [21] concept, is a framework for staging ARF based on "susceptibility" derived from epidemiologic studies, "insult" based on the knowledge of the specific insult and the time interval from the insult to the point of evaluation, "response" after the RIFLE criteria, and "outcome" [22]; however, this concept has yet to be validated.

Outcome prediction scores such as APACHE II or SAPS II have been used for AKI prediction, but more specific scores to predict outcome for patients with ARF in the ICU have been developed, for example, those designed by Liaño and colleagues (ISI) [23] or the Cleveland Clinic [24]. The exact role of these scales in this setting has not been definitely proved. In our experience, the SOFA score was a better predictor of outcome in ICU patients with ARF than the ISI score and others [6].

4
Diagnosis and Monitoring

4.1
Conventional Biomarkers for AKI

The most useful parameter for evaluating renal function is the GFR; however, in clinical practice it is not measured but estimated. Creatinine clearance has become the standard in clinics for estimating GFR, but it is cumbersome and not widely used. Serum Cr_s is an indirect reflection of GFR when renal function is in a steady state and is the most widely used estimate for GFR. One of the main problems with Cr_s, namely, being a "static" measure and being delayed after GFR (Fig. 1), is somewhat overcome by its inclusion in a multilevel "dynamic" classification such as the already mentioned RIFLE or AKIN classifications.

Table 2 AKIN classification [20]

Group	Glomerular filtration rate criteria	Urine output criteria
1	↑ Cr_s of >0.3 mg dL^{-1} or increase to ≥150% – 200% (1.5–2 fold) from baseline	<0.5 mL kg^{-1} h^{-1} for >6 h
2	↑ Cr_s to >200–300% (>2–3 fold) from baseline	<0.5 mL kg^{-1} h^{-1} for >12 h
3	↑ Cr_s to >300% (>3 fold) from baseline (or Cr_s ≥4.0 mg dL^{-1} with an acute rise of at least 0.5 mg dL^{-1})	<0.3 mL kg^{-1} h^{-1} × 24 h or anuria × 12 h

Cr_s serum creatinine

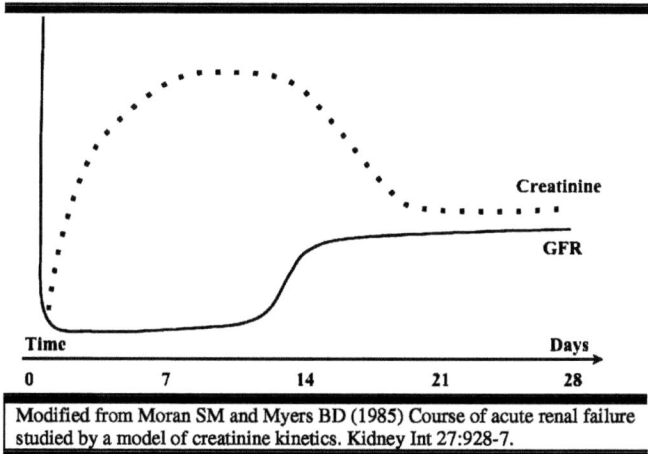

Fig. 1 Relationship between glomerular filtration rate and serum creatinine (modified from [95])

Table 3 Early biomarkers for detecting AKI [27]

Biomarker	Origin	Clinical implications
Tubular enzymes	Brush border	Early detection
Low molecular weight proteins	Glomerular filtration	Need for depuration
NHE-3	Na+ transporter	Not present in prerenal states
NGAL	Concentrated in proximal tubule after ischemia	Sensible for ischemia
CYR61	Heparin binding protein, expression after medular insults	Early in ischemia
IL-6-8-18	In proximal tubular cells (IL-18 potentiates ischemia)	Early in ischemia
KIM-1	Tubular membrane protein expressed after ischemia	FRA development
Perforins	Cytotoxic proteins	Rejection after transplant
Endothelins	Endothelin-like in urine	After radio contrast

4.2
New Biomarkers for AKI

In diagnosing AKI, our ultimate goal should be to define sensitive and specific biomarkers, capable of detecting AKI in the early stages in order to prevent the evolution to overt ARF (and improve the prognosis) (Table 3) [25]. Recently, a molecule known to appear after ischemic insults (KIM-1) was isolated in the urine of ANT patients, which could aid in the early detection of AKI [26]. Another possible marker is the Na^+/H^+ exchanger isoform ($NHE3^+$) that was specific for ATN in a study comparing patients with AKI against control subjects [27]. The neutrophil gelatinase-associated lipocalin (NGAL) was tested in children after cardiac surgery and showed an area under the curve of 0.998 for detecting AKI [28], but these good results could not be reproduced in adult patients. Other molecules tested but not yet validated are Cyr68, perforins, or interleukins 6–8 or 18. Unfortunately we are far from having the ideal marker for septic AKI and the ones that have been tested are inadequate, inherently inconsistent, and limited by a multiplicity of factors, including study design, no inclusion of septic patients, and numerous confounding variables [29].

Cystatine-C (Cys-C) is very useful because of its potential benefits and the experience accumulated. Cys-C is produced at a constant rate and is not related to age, sex, or muscular mass and is completely reabsorbed at the tubules. It seems to be more exact than Cr_s as a surrogate of GRF [30–32]. Another important advantage is its precocity; Cys-C can detect renal dysfunction 1 or 2 days before Cr_s increases [33]. A recent meta-analysis points to Cys-C as a better marker of GFR than Cr_s [34]. Cys-C seems to be a promising tool, but we need more data before its place in the detection of AKI is definitely settled.

4.3
Monitoring and Diagnostic Tests

In addition to blood urea nitrogen (BUN) and *creatinine*, there are some diagnostic tools that could be helpful for diagnosing and monitoring patients with impairment of renal function at the bedside. As mentioned previously, Cr_s (filtered in the glomerulus without resorption, metabolism, or tubular secretion) forms the basis of the diagnosis and monitoring of AKI. We should specify that a proportion of creatinine is secreted in the renal tubule (10%), which leads to an overestimation of the real GFR in ClCr calculation. It has an exponential growth; with a loss of 50% of nephrons, the GFR decreases 50%, but Cr_s does not reach pathological states. Up to this point, a small loss of parenchymal function may cause high creatinine levels. Well-known experts in the field defend this parameter as the main one in acute renal function worsening [15].

Agreement has been reached on the estimated *glomerular filtration rate* (GFR) being the parameter with which to recognize renal function. The only issue is the difficulty of measuring it at the bedside [23]. Beside Cr_s measurement, CrCl is one of the basic diagnostic and monitoring tools for estimating GFR. Measuring CrCl in a short time span (2 h) was demonstrated by Herrera-Gutierrez et al. [35] to be a good method (easy to perform and closely related to the standard 24-h measurement) for estimation of GFR in the ICU. The use of equations to estimate GFR in ICU patients has not been validated and the scarce data published preclude their use in this setting [36].

Ultrasonography (US), as a minimally invasive tool, should play the leading role in the differential diagnosis of AKI [37] and sepsis-related AKI. Some findings show chronic renal failure: small and hypoechogenic kidneys, big bilateral renal cysts, and reduced renal parenchyma. In urologic and retroperitoneal surgery this tool is very useful for diagnosing postrenal AKI. When there is AKI and US does not show abnormalities, we should go further into the diagnostic algorithm.

Fractional excretion of sodium (FENa) (Na$_{urine}$ × Creatinine$_{plasma}$)/(Na$_{plasma}$ × Creatinine$_{urine}$) in percentage is another functional test that helps in the diagnosis and treatment of AKI. Scores over 1 or 3% point to intrinsic renal failure (parenchymatous damage). On the other hand, an *FENa* less than 1% shows decreased effective circulating volume (cardiac failure, hypovolemia, hepatorenal syndrome) without intrinsic parenchymatous damage. This parameter is not useful for patients managed with diuretics, because sodium secretion is altered.

The differential diagnosis between functional and intrinsic kidney injury may be completed with information from Table 4.

Renal biopsy [37] in septic AKI patients should be done when an etiology other than acute tubular necrosis is suspected (e.g., small vessel vasculitis, glomerulonephritis, interstitial inmunoallergic nephritis, amyloidosis etc.).

Diagnostic Algorithm: In summary, we should base the diagnostic approach to AKI on establishing whether it is an acute injury (clinical history +/− US), ruling out postrenal AKI (US), and finally differentiating between a prerenal situation and a parenchymatous AKI (clinical history, laboratory results +/− biopsy).

5
AKI Prevention

5.1
Ischemic Renal Failure

Prophylaxis is based on *optimizing renal perfusion*, depending on a good renal blood flow and intrarenal distribution of this flow. Cardiac output, mean arterial pressure, and glomerular hemodynamics (afferent and efferent arteriole) are key hemodynamic issues. Although the kidneys represent only 1% of body weight, they receive around 25% of cardiac output, being the best perfused tissue, essential for the body's proper functioning. Drops in cardiac output not only decrease renal blood flow, but neurohormonal vasoconstriction mechanisms are also activated. Any action to restore cardiac output will improve renal flow, and giving intravenous fluids to hypovolemic patients is the most accurate action in preventing septic AKI. Some investigators tend to doubt the improvement in the prognosis of critically ill patients when monitored; however, we agree with other authors that monitoring devices are as good as the doctor in interpreting the results, and we think it is necessary to pay attention to learning and improving clinical practice with these monitoring devices. We should add

Table 4 Distinguishing findings between prerenal disease and renal ischemic damage (acute tubular necrosis, ATN)

Measurement	Prerenal disease	Renal damage (ATN)
Urine osmolality	>500	<400
Urine sodium	<20	>40
Urine creatinine/plasmatic creatinine	>40	<20
FENa (%)	<1	>2
Urine sediment	Granular	Epithelial cells

that there is a study on critically ill patients with AKI where pulmonary artery catheter (PAC) insertion at the time of study inclusion was related to a better outcome as an independent factor [38]. Some other measurements like central venous pressure and mixed venous saturation have proved effective in predicting a better outcome in critically ill patients [39]. It is well known that improvement in outcome is related to a proper intravascular resuscitation, although fluid overloading may become a hazard [40]. Restrictive strategies in fluid therapy may also improve respiratory function without harm to other organs or systems, for example, the kidneys [41]. The knowledge on AKI prevention invite to manage haemodynamic based on general clinical practice. For this approach we should choose the best-known monitoring device aiming for isovolemia and avoiding hypervolemia.

Regarding the deleterious effect of hemodynamic worsening on renal tissue, *intra-abdominal hypertension* (IAH) has been recognized as a risk factor for AKI since 1990. Although abdominal pressures over 15 mmHg have been experimentally related to AKI, values over 10 mmHg may cause worsening in GFR. A recent study set pressures of 12 mmHg as an independent risk factor in AKI, although the authors stress the value of the hemodynamic state of the patient: shock and abdominal perfusion pressure (APP) [42]. The Word Society of Abdominal Compartment Syndrome (WSACS) also chose 12 mmHg standing values as indicative of IAH and defined abdominal compartment syndrome (ACS) standing values of IAP over 20 mmHg, with or without APP of 60 mmHg, with a new organ dysfunction. It is important to enhance how AKI can play a double role as cause and consequence [43, 44]. ACS must be noted and treated in order to prevent AKI.

To avoid iatrogenia in *glomerular hemodynamics* (afferent and efferent arteriole) we should consider the common drugs we use that affect glomerular autoregulation: nonsteroidal anti-inflammatory drugs and angiotensin-converting enzyme inhibitors [45]. When intravascular volume is reduced there is an increase in renin and angiotensin release that causes renal vasoconstriction. In such situations, prostaglandins play an important role against vasoconstriction. Nonsteroidal anti-inflammatory drugs reduce prostaglandin synthesis, decreasing glomerular filtration speed and renal flow, especially when intravascular volume is reduced. In the afferent arteriole, inhibition of angiotensin-converting enzyme can block vasoconstriction that maintains glomerular filtration pressure. Thus, angiotensin-converting enzyme inhibitors could deteriorate prerenal AKI due to the vasoconstriction of the afferent arteriole.

5.2
Toxic Renal Failure

Although many drugs have renal toxic effects, we will pay attention to aminoglycosides and radiocontrast agents, which have specific prevention protocols and are difficult to substitute by less toxic molecules.

Aminoglycosides: The incidence of AKI secondary to aminoglycosides is between 5 and 50% during long-standing treatments. Renal toxicity is produced along the proximal tubule. Early diagnosis can be made by analyzing urine deposits with an increased concentration of proteins, leukocytes, and cylinders. It is well known that aminoglycosides given once a day decrease renal toxicity, maintaining an antimicrobial effect [46].

Radiocontrasts: Changes in renal function occur 48 h after administration of radiocontrast material [47]. The worst values of creatinine are found between the third and the fifth day and some patients may develop nephropathy 1 week after the contrast agent was given. This is the third cause of AKI in Europe and the United States. Despite progress in this area, the number of contrast-induced AKI cases keeps rising. Although the mechanisms involved are not well known, there are two events taking place: direct nephrotoxic effect and secondary intrarenal vasoconstriction. These effects are less frequent with low osmolality contrast agents such as iodixanol [47].

Although it is proved that isotonic contrast agents are less nephrotoxic, we should restrict their use to high-risk patients due to the high costs. To find the best candidates for isotonic contrast agents, we may stratify patients following the guidelines presented in Table 5, where values equal to or less than 5 show low risks for contrast-induced nephropathy.

The second step to avoid is administration of drugs that could boost any nephrotoxic effects. *Metformin* should be stopped 24 h before radiocontrast administration and reintroduced 48 h later [48], otherwise it can induce lactic acidosis (8%) and AKI (4%). *Nephrotoxic antibiotics* should also be avoided due to their additive nephrotoxic effect. *Nonsteroidal anti-inflammatory drugs* increase contrast-induced disturbances in experimental models. New cox-2 inhibitors do not offer real advantage. *Dipyridamole* induces an increase in adenosine. Since a rise in adenosine is decisive in nephrotoxicity, dipyridamole should not be use in such circumstances.

Angiotensin-Converting Enzyme Inhibitors: The latest consensus recommendations [48] for contrast-induced nephropathy recommend not starting to give these drugs before contrast administration, but not to stop them if the patient was already under treatment.

Finally, the value of avoiding a reduced *circulating effective volume* should be emphasized, since it is another important risk factor in contrast-related nephrotoxicity. Previous hemodynamic optimization and iso-osmolar rehydration (with saline or bicarbonate) have been demonstrated to lower the rate of contrast-related nephrotoxicity [49].

Table 5 Contrast-induced nephropathy risk score (modified from [38])

Variable	Points
Hypotension (SBP < 80 mmHg during 1 h at least)	5
Intra-aortic balloon pump within 24 h peri-procedurally	5
Congestive cardiac failure (III/IV AHA classification)	4
Age >75 years	4
Serum creatinine >1.5 mg dL^{-1}	4
Glomerular filtration rate <20 mL min^{-1} 1.73 m^2	6
Glomerular filtration rate 20–40 mL min^{-1} 1.73 m^2	4
Glomerular filtration rate 40–60 mL min^{-1} 1.73 m^2	2
Anemia (hematocrit <39% for men and <36% for women)	3
Diabetes mellitus	3
Volume of contrast (every 100 ml of contrast)	1

In several studies, *N*-acetylcysteine demonstrated its efficiency and strength in the prophylaxis of CRN (Contrast-Related Nephrotoxicity), but it should not take the place of hemodynamic optimization [49]. The recommended oral dose is 600 mg 12 h^{-1} during 24 h before and after exposition. The optimal intravenous dose is still to be determined.

5.3
Other Preventive Actions

Dopamine: It is currently well known that dopamine does not prevent AKI or decrease the risk of extracorporeal purification blood treatments or death in patients with AKI, and therefore using this drug as a therapeutic tool is considered bad clinical practice [50].

Fenoldopam: This selective agonist of dopamine-1 receptor increases renal flow. After negative results in several studies, it was recently shown in a clinical trial that long-term administration (10 days) of fenoldopam decreased AKI in critically ill patients, on top if its hypotensive effect.

Hemofiltration. A single-center and biased study (no standardized hydration regime, no use of iso-osmolar contrast and comparison between critically ill patients and ward patients) concluded that more evidence is needed on hemofiltration before it can be recommended as a first-line tool in the prophylaxis of contrast-related nephrotoxicity [49].

Loop Diuretics and Mannitol: Although it is well accepted by doctors caring for critically ill patients that loop diuretics and mannitol improve diuresis, there is no evidence of any positive effect on AKI, and since there are several negative effects, they should be used only for the treatment of hypervolemic states.

6
Management

6.1
General Management

In sepsis-related ARF, the first step is to treat sepsis. Restoring hemodynamics as soon as possible and continuing with prophylaxis are also priorities [11]. AKI is per se an independent factor for outcome of multiorgan dysfunction syndrome (MODS), but the prognosis of AKI is closely related to the evolution of MODS [7].

When AKI progresses, some renal functions need to be replaced by extracorporeal treatments.

6.2
Renal Replacement Therapies

In this section we discuss the way to perform blood purification by extracorporeal treatments and their influence on outcome in patients with AKI and with MODS.

6.2.1
General Considerations for Renal Replacement Therapy

The objective of extracorporeal treatment in AKI is different to that of chronic renal failure, in which we try to delay as much as possible the initiation of extracorporeal purification treatments (EPT). In AKI, we try to minimize "metabolic" complications that can affect negatively the evolution of the patient; hence, in this clinical context the approaches regarding "dosage" of chronically ill patients are not necessarily applicable. We prefer to speak about "renal support" instead of renal replacement therapy (RRT).

Conventional intermittent hemodialysis (IHD) frequently presents many problems when used for this type of patient, often having a limited ability to reduce volume because of the patient-associated hemodynamic instability and hypotension. In 1977 Kramer et al. described the continuous arteriovenous hemofiltration technique, which was the first continuous renal replacement therapy (CRRT). Today modern modalities allow a more accurate and effective control of the plasmatic urea and intravascular volume without the need for staff especially trained in hemodialysis therapy [51]. The slow and continuous ultrafiltration rate of the CRRT avoids the rapid shifts in intravascular volume and electrolyte concentrations that are seen with IHD. However, CRRT is not exempt from inconveniences. A longer period of blood contact with strange material involves more possibilities of inflammatory reaction, as well as a greater necessity for anticoagulation. Additionally, it could bear higher costs for treatment, being mainly based on liquids (reposition and dialysis).

6.2.2
Renal Replacement Therapy and Acute Renal Failure

IHD treatment is usually offered to hemodynamically unstable AKI patients, who usually present with severe hypotension and cardiac dysrhythmias, which along with tissular ischemia (because of hypotension) and the need for volume restriction (because of the nutrition volume requirements) limit the patient management [52]. CRRT allows the removal of almost any volume of fluid over a 24-h period without sudden shifts in the patient intravascular volume.

Several studies support the usefulness of continuous techniques in AKI patients, even in those with a high catabolic profile [53, 54]. Although there is no question about the fluid removal capability of these techniques, the amount of solute clearance required to achieve an optimal metabolic control of the patient remains less clear. Some studies that initiated prophylactic dialysis suggested that lowering plasmatic urea nitrogen below 100–120 mg dL^{-1} improves survival in AKI patients [53]. CRRTs present several advantages when they are compared with IHD, and they are generally considered the techniques of choice for the treatment of AKI in critically unstable patients. However, although they facilitate greatly the handling of these patients, it has not been demonstrated clearly whether these techniques improve the survival. Several studies have compared the evolution of patients with AKI treated with IHD or with CRRT [55, 56]. In one of the most important meta-analyses published [57], which compared patients with a similar level of severity in the studies carried out to date (13 studies, with 1,400 patients), it was found that the decrease in hospital mortality with CRRT was clearly significant ($p < 0.01$). Moreover, it was demonstrated that there is a significantly better and faster recovery of AKI when CRRT is used [57, 58]. When patients are not distributed according to the level of severity, as in the meta-analysis carried out by Bagshaw and colleagues [59], there are no differences in outcome among patients, although the hemodynamic tolerance seems to be better with CRRT.

Although it is clear that the most critically ill patients benefit from CRRT, some authors [60] only find benefit in serious, but not "excessively" critically ill patients, thereby selecting even more the patient "type" to benefit from CRRT.

Of the most recent controlled studies [61–63], the one that has raised the biggest interest and controversy has been that of Vinsonneau (360 multicenter patients). In this study, no differences in mortality were found when comparing various therapeutic techniques; however, when the work is analyzed it is appreciated that the CRRT used is very conservative compared with an intermittent "exquisite" technique, with an increase in the frequency of sessions during the study.

Two recent large multicenter trials, ATN and RENAL [63] (the RENAL trial is still ongoing), which compare in a controlled way an intensive treatment with a conventional one for stable and unstable patients, have selected extended techniques over time for unstable patients. It seems that, in spite of the apparent controversy, when studies are designed using unstable patients the profitability of intermittent techniques is overlooked.

We should not forget that there are hybrid techniques available that could have a place in some scenarios. The idea of making the intermittent techniques more "continuous" has led some groups to develop SLEDD ("slow low-efficient daily dialysis"), which could be useful in certain contexts. It consists of an IHD carried out with a low flow of blood and dialysis liquid, over more time (6–12 h/day) [64]. This technique offers greater hemodynamic stability, better correction of the hypervolemia, and a more appropriate metabolic control than the intermittent classic techniques.

Regarding the "dosage" of EPT, several "classic" studies seem to point toward the idea that a greater quantity of dialysis treatment (Kt/V for session or bigger number of sessions) contributed to greater survival.

It seems that a greater quantity of purification is correlated with an improvement in outcome. The classic work of Ronco and colleagues [65], in a prospective randomized study, demonstrated in a group of 425 critically ill patients with AKI that, when using polysulfone membranes, the hemofiltrate volume schedule should be up to 35 mL kg^{-1}, thereby achieving a significant reduction in mortality ($p < 0.0007$) in the 15 days of having suspended EPT. This principle (more dose = better outcome) is also extended to IHD. Schiffl and coworkers [66] demonstrated a better survival and recovery of AKI when the conventional dialysis was carried out on a daily basis instead of with the classic alternating schedule. This work has been criticized because the authors used a low dose (Kt/V of 0.94) per session, and therefore the treatment dose for the alternating-days group would have been inferior to the one normally used.

The recently published multicenter ATN study [67] failed to show a beneficial effect of higher doses of RRT on the survival of AKI patients or the rate of recovery of kidney function or nonrenal organ failure. In this elegant study 1,124 critically ill patients with AKI and failure of at least one nonrenal organ or sepsis were randomized to receive intensive or less intensive RRT. Interestingly, in both study groups, hemodynamically stable patients underwent intermittent hemodialysis, and hemodynamically unstable patients underwent continuous venovenous hemodiafiltration (CVVHF) or sustained low-efficiency dialysis.

A recent publication [68] presents the different comments and limitations outlined by some authors regarding the study. It is emphasized that the study's own authors recognize that their results do not imply that the dose is not important. The limitations of the study are the different inclusion criteria and clinical results to those previously published. We find of special relevance the fact that the half-stay in hospital at the time of inclusion was 10.3–11.1 days and in the ICU 6.4–6.9 days. This does not include in the analysis the first week of stay in the ICU, which could be important since data exist in the literature suggesting that the impact of these treatments can be related to early use [69, 70] and that it is in these phases that a certain dose can have more impact on the hemodynamic state [71].

The results should invite us to contemplate whether maintaining the same dose of purification during the entire treatment course of a critical patient is appropriate or not.

Some authors recommend adjusting the purification dose according to the severity of the patients [66, 72], maintaining that the benefits related with larger or smaller doses are found in a subgroup of patients who are neither too healthy nor near death. This approach for different patients could be accepted. The clinical evolution of a critically ill patient is dynamic, from critically ill to subacute illness. Therefore, it is difficult to assume that the necessities of the purification dose are the same during the entire duration of a patient's ICU stay. This dynamic dose pattern that is recommended for patients with different severity [66] should also be outlined, in our opinion, to an individual patient that shows changes in diseases severity over time [73], following the diagram presented in Fig. 2. Aspects such as compensation of the loss of valuable substances (ions, nutrition, drugs, etc.) and handling of the

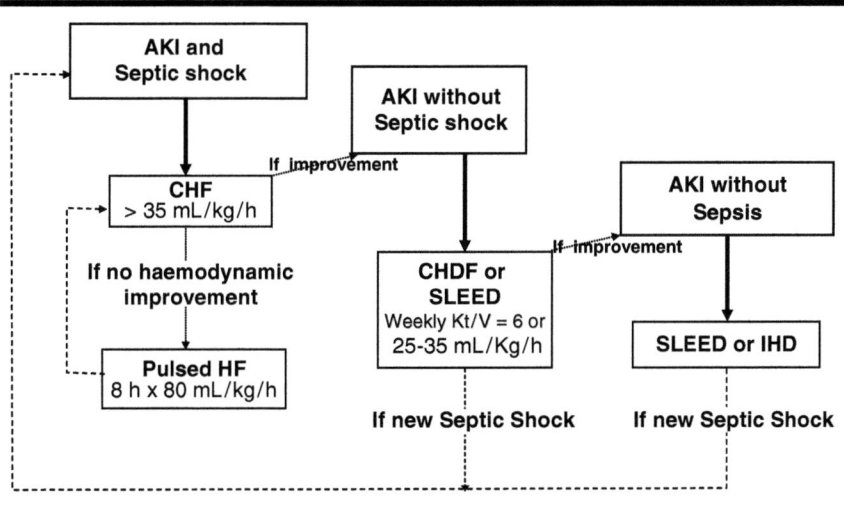

Fig. 2 Diagram of a dynamic approach to extracorporeal purification treatments for AKI based on different clinical status. Intermittent modalities imply that periods without treatments are well tolerated by patient in terms of fluid balance and general homeostasis. Otherwise, continuous regimen must be used. *AKI* acute kidney injury, *C* continuous, *HF* hemofiltration, *SLEED* slow low efficiency extended dialysis, *HDF* hemodiafiltration, *IHD* intermittent hemodialysis

fluid balance are also important for the evaluation of results. All these problems are encompassed in the term "dialytrauma" [73], which includes the associated morbidity to a bad dosage of EPT that one can recognize in the patient as: hypopotasemia, hypophosphoremia, hypothermia, bleeding related to the chosen anticoagulation regime, etc.

We will need to wait for the final results of the RENAL study to get more information on the importance of the dosage being adapted in this particular type of therapy and particular type of patient.

Another aspect that is gaining importance in the last few years is the possibility of giving an appropriate purification dose combining convection and diffusion [72, 74]. The diffusion use prolongs the survival of the CRRT circuits [75], which has obvious benefits.

The time of initiation of the RRT also plays an important role in the ARF patient's outcome. Currently the term "renal support" is preferred to the classic term "renal replacement therapy" [53], supporting an earlier initiation of renal replacement [65].

There are fewer data available on ending treatment, although we can recommend the approaches proposed by Ronco and Bellomo [54] that are quite logical: diuresis >1 mL kg^{-1} h^{-1} for >24 h; possibility of neutral hydric balance, without reduction of the necessary volume; absence of complications of uremia. We recommend carrying out a weaning test as done in other treatments. If the patient is able to maintain homeostasis and fluid balance without CRRT, we would end the treatment definitively.

6.2.3
Sepsis and MODS

There are data suggesting that CRRT can influence the clinical evolution of MODS patients, improving their outcome even in the absence of renal failure [76].

Our experience supports these results. In a first study [77], we prospectively analyzed the effect of 12 h of CVVHF on the hemodynamic profile and respiratory function of 55 critically ill patients with MODS; 35 of these patients presented with anuric AKI. Hemofiltration significantly improved several hemodynamic and respiratory parameters. In a former prospective, randomized, controlled study, we analyzed the effects of CVVHF on the hemodynamic and respiratory function of a group of severely traumatized patients with incipient MODS but without AKI. The evaluation period was prolonged to 48 h. CVVHF significantly improved MAP (Mean Arterial Pressure) values ($p = 0.0001$) without having any effects on central venous pressure, PAOP (Pulmonary Artery Occlusion Pressure), or cardiac output. We also found a clear improvement in oxygenation and ventilation in CRRT patients. In the context of MODS, several studies in animal models have confirmed a correlation between survival and ultrafiltration rate [78].

In humans, Oudemans-Van Straaten and colleagues [79] analyzed the results obtained from 306 patients (52% oliguric). They found a significantly lower observed mortality than predicted mortality in the CRRT group, based on the APACHE II, SAPS II, and the index of Liaño. Honoré and coworkers [69] tested a cycle of high-volume hemofiltrate (35 l, in 4 h), followed by at least 4 days of conventional hemofiltrate (1 l/h). They defined a group of 11 patients as "responders," based on the improvement of cardiac index, the positive evolution of the acidemia, and the drop in inotropic drug requirements. The mortality in this group was only of 18%. The global observed mortality was inferior to the one predicted based on APACHE II ($p < 0.05$). They observed that the "responders" group was subjected to CRRT earlier and with a higher dose than the "nonresponders" group.

Another recent study [71] analyzed the evolution of hemodynamics and that of several inflammatory mediators in a group of patients with septic shock and MODS who were randomly subjected to an 8-h cycle of a high-volume hemofiltration (6 L h^{-1}) or a cycle of 8 h of conventional (1 L h^{-1}) hemofiltrate. The authors found that both techniques improved significantly the hemodynamics of these patients (decrease in the dose of noradrenaline) and lowered the concentration of several of the inflammatory mediators analyzed. The technique of high-volume hemofiltration accentuates these positive effects.

Joannes-Boyau and coworkers [80] applied hemofiltration volumes of 40–60 mL kg^{-1} h^{-1} over 96 h to a group of patients in septic shock, and saw a significant improvement in hemodynamics of the 24 patients, as well as an improvement in the observed mortality ($p < 0.075$) versus predicted mortality using three different severity scores.

Ratanarat and colleagues [81] analyzed the effect of a technique consisting in a high-volume "pulse" of 6–8 h of replacement of 85 mL kg^{-1} h^{-1} followed by 16–18 h with a volume of 35 mL kg^{-1} h^{-1} in 15 patients with serious sepsis. These authors found a clear hemodynamic benefit and an improvement in the predicted survival.

More recently, Piccinni et al. [82] analyzed the effect of high-volume hemofiltration (45 mL kg^{-1} h^{-1}) applied early (first 12 h) to septic shock patients. In a retrospective study of 80 critically ill patients (40 of them with conventional treatment and 40 with a new protocol of precocious hemofiltrate), the effect of this high volume was analyzed for 6 h, followed by a conventional hemofiltration technique. The authors observed a significant improvement in hemodynamics and breathing, as well as in the survival, after setting-up the new protocol.

In other contexts of MODS, very good results have been achieved in experiences with serious acute pancreatitis and extra-hospital heart arrest [59–65].

Some authors [78] have proposed a detailed classification for HVHF, maintaining the dose from 35 to 50 mL kg^{-1} h^{-1}, as with the critical patient's "renal" dose, but introducing a "dose for septic patients" (more than 50 mL kg^{-1} h^{-1}) and a "dose for serious hemodynamic instability" (100–215 mL kg^{-1} h^{-1}).

6.2.4
Putative Mechanisms for Effectiveness in Sepsis and MODS

With these clinically consistent results, the most widely accepted hypothesis to explain them is the one based on the immunomodulatory ability of these therapies.

The convective elimination of several inflammatory mediators with RRT is an accepted fact in animal models and in clinical experience with humans. On the other hand, although inflammatory mediators can be in the filtrate, it still needs to be demonstrated that this elimination produces a significant decrease in their plasma levels.

In this way, multiple authors have confirmed the utility of CRRT in the "significant" elimination of several inflammatory mediators [83–86].

With this body of evidence, the potential benefits of EPT are explained with the "peak concentration hypothesis" [87] according to which, the increase in convection and other depurative mechanisms immunomodulate the sepsis. Only the studies by Yekebas on serious acute pancreatitis [88] have been able to reproduce this hypothesis. Our clinical randomized study on traumatic patients [89] could have the same interpretation, with a decrease in distal cytokines of the inflammatory cascade. Tromboxane-A2 was diminished significantly in the treatment group, and the evolution of leukotriene-B4 almost reached statistical significance.

6.2.5
Controversial Aspects of HVHF

When considering to use such high clearing rates, some controversial issues surface.

We should not forget the important adsorptive capacity of some membranes, able to eliminate significant quantities of cytokines [71]. The possibility to use membranes with a bigger pore [90] could also affect the ability of eliminating biologically active substances.

Lastly, the possibility to eliminate valuable substances should be approached with caution when introducing these techniques in the clinic. Any molecule with a low molecular weight (lower than 40 kDa), with an elevated fraction not fixed to proteins and a low distribution volume, can be eliminated significantly with these techniques. This includes most of the drugs used today (more than 90% of the antibiotics, for example) and a multitude of nutrients [91–94]. These losses must be balanced, or the treatments will worsen the so-called dialytrauma [73].

References

1. Hank WK, Bonventie JV (2004) Biologic markers for the early detection of acute kidney injury. Curr Opin Crit Care 10:476–482
2. Kellum JA, Levin N, Bouman C, Lameire N (2002) Developing a consensus classification system for acute renal failure. Curr Opin Crit Care 8:509–514
3. Shusterman N, Strom BL, Murray TG, Morrison G, West SL, Maislin G (1987) Risk factors and outcome of hospital-acquired acute renal failure. Am J Med 83:65–71
4. Levy EM, Viscoli CM, Horwitz RI (1996) The effect of acute renal failure on mortality: A cohort analysis. JAMA 75:1489–1494
5. Liaño F, Junco E, Pascual J, Madero R, Verde E (1998) The spectrum of acute renal failure in the intensive care unit compared with that seen in other settings. The Madrid Acute Renal Failure Study Group. Kidney Int 66:S16–S24
6. Herrera ME, Seller G, Maynar J, Sánchez-Izquierdo JA, et al. (2006) Epidemiología del FRA en las UCI españolas: Estudio prospectivo multicéntrico FRAMI. Med Intensiva 30:260–267
7. Maynar J, Corral E, Gainza J, et al. (1997) Acute renal failure in critically ill patients: a descriptive, prospective multicenter study. Preliminary results [Abstract]. Intens Care Med 23:S142
8. Uchino S, Kellum JA, Bellomo R, Doig GS, Morimatsu H, et al., for the beginning and ending supportive therapy for the kidney (BEST Kidney) investigators (2005) Acute Renal Failure in Critically Ill Patients A Multinational, Multicenter Study. JAMA 294:813–818
9. Brivet FG, Kleinknecht DJ, Loirat P, Landais PJ (1996) Acute renal failure in intensive care units: Causes, outcome, and prognostic factors of hospital mortality – A prospective, multicenter study. French Study Group on Acute Renal Failure. Crit Care Med 24:192–198
10. Schrier RW, Wang W (2004) Acute renal failure and sepsis. N Engl J Med 351:159–169

11. Hoste EA, Lameire NH, Vanholder RC, et al. (2003) Acute renal failure in patients with sepsis in a surgical ICU: Predictive factors, incidence, comorbidity, and outcome. J Am Soc Nephrol 14:1022–1030
12. Riedemann NC, Guo RF, Ward PA (2003) The enigma of sepsis. J Clin Invest 112:460–467
13. Hoste EA, Clermont G, Kersten A, Venkataraman R, Angus DC, et al. (2006) RIFLE criteria for acute kidney injury are associated with hospital mortality in critically ill patients: a cohort análisis. Critical Care 10:R73
14. Ricci Z, Ronco C, D'amico G, et al. (2006) Practice patterns in the management of acute renal failure in the critically ill patient: an international survey. Nephrol Dial Transplant 21:690–696
15. Bellomo R, Ronco C, Kellum JA, ADQI workgroup (2004) Acute renal failure: definition, outcome measures, animal models, fluid therapy and information technology needs: the second international consensus conference of the Acute Dialysis Quality Initiative (ADQI) Group. Crit Care Med 8:204–212
16. Ostermann M, Chang RWS (2007) Acute kidney injury in the intensive care unit according to RIFLE. Crit Care Med 35:1837–1843
17. Herrera ME, Seller G, Banderas E Moreno J, Lebrón M, Quesada J (2008) Diferencias en la clasificación de pacientes usando la escala RIFLE según el parámetro de estimación de GFR empleado [Abstract]. Med Intensiva 32:22
18. Lassnigg A, Schmidlin D, Mouhieddine M, Bachmann LM, Druml W, et al. (2004) Minimal changes of serum creatinine predict prognosis in patients alter cardiothoracic surgery: a prospective cohort study. J Am Soc Nephrol 15:1597–1605
19. Chertow GM, Burdick E, Honour M, et al. (2005) Acute kidney injury, mortality, length of stay, and costs in hospitalized patients. J Am Soc Nephrol 16:3365–3370
20. Mehta RL, Kellum JA, Shah SV, Molitoris BA, Ronco C, Warnock DG, Levin A (2007) Acute Kidney Injury Network: report of an initiative to improve outcomes in acute kidney injury; Acute Kidney Injury Network. Critical Care 11:R31
21. Levy MM, Fink MP, Marshall JC, Abraham E, Angus D, Cook D, Cohen J, Opal SM, Vincent JL, Ramsay G (2003) International Sepsis Definitions Conference. 2001 SCCM/ESICM/ACCP/ATS/SIS International Sepsis Definitions Conference. Intens Care Med 29:530–538
22. Mehta R, Chertow GM (2003) Acute renal failure definitions and classification: time for change? J Am Soc Nephrol 14:2178–2187
23. Liaño F, Gallego A, Pascual J, et al. (1993) Prognosis of ATN: an extended prospectively contrasted study. Nephron 63:21–31
24. Douma CE, Redekop WK, Van Den Meulen JHP, et al. (1997) Predicting mortality in ICU patients with ARF treated with dialysis. J Am Soc Nephrol 8:111–117
25. Trof RJ, Di Maggio F, Leemreis J, Groeneveld J (2006) Biomarkers of acute renal injury and renal failure. Shock 26:245–253
26. Han WK, Bailly V, Abichandani R, et al. (2002) Kidney injury molecule-1 (KIM-1): a novel biomarker for human renal proximal tubule injury. Kidney Int 62:237–244
27. Cheyron D, Daubin C, Poggioli J, et al. (2003) Urinary measurement of Na_/H_ exchanger isoform 3 (NHE3) protein as new marker of tubule injury in critically ill patients with ARF. Am J Kidney Dis 42:497–506
28. Wagener G, Jan M, Kim M, Mori K, Barasch JM, Sladen RN, Lee HT (2006) Association between increases in urinary neutrophil gelatinase-associated lipocalin and acute renal dysfunction after adult cardiac surgery. Anesthesiology 105:485–491
29. Bagshaw SM, Langenberg C, Bellomo R (2006) Urinary biochemistry and microscopy in septic acute renal failure: A systematic review. Am J Kidney Dis 48:695–705
30. Villa P, Jiménez M, Soriano MC, et al. (2005) Serum cystatin C concentration as a marker of acute renal dysfunction in critically ill patients. Crit Care 9:R139–R143
31. Delanaye P, Lambermont B, Chapelle JP, et al. (2004) Plasmatic cystatin C for the estimation of glomerular filtration rate in intensive care units. Intens Care Med 30:980–983

32. Le Bricon T, Leblanc I, Benlakehal M, et al. (2005) Evaluation of renal function in intensive care: plasma cyctatin C vs. creatinine and derived glomerular filtration rate stimates. Clin Chem Lab Med 43:953–957
33. Knight EL, Verhave JC, Spielgelman D, et al. (2004) Factors influencing serum cystatin C levels other than renal function and the impact on renal function measurement. Kidney Int 65:1416–1421
34. Dharnidharka VR, Kwon C, Stevens G (2002) Serum cystatin C is superior to serum creatinine as a marker of kidney function: A meta-analysis. Am J Kidney Dis 40:221–226
35. Herrera ME, Seller G, Banderas E, Muñoz J, Lebrón M, Fernández F (2007) Replacement of 24-h creatinine clearance by 2-h creatinine clearance in intensive care unit patients: a single-center study. Intens Care Med 33:1900–1906
36. Seller G, Herrera ME, Banderas E Moreno J, Lebrón M, Muñoz J (2007) Utilidad de las fórmulas de Cockroft-Gault y Jeliffe para calcular el aclaramiento de creatinina en UCI [Abstract]. Med Intensiva 31:42
37. Maynar J y Sánchez-Izquierdo JA (2001) Editores de la Monografía. Fallo Renal Agudo y Técnicas de Reemplazo Renal. Barcelona. EDIKAMED. ISBN 84-7877-290-1
38. Uchino S, Doig GS, Bellomo R, et al. (2004) Diuretics and mortality in acute renal failure. Crit Care Med 32:1669–1677
39. Rivers M, Nguyen B, Havstad S, et al. (2001) Early goal-directed therapy in the treatment of severe sepsis and septic shock. N Engl J Med 345:1368–1377
40. Vincent J-L Sakr Y, Sprun CL (2006) Sepsis in European intensive care units: Results of the SOAP study. Crit Care Med 34:344–353
41. The National Heart, Lung, and Blood Institute Acute Respiratory Distress Syndrome (ARDS) Clinical Trials Network. (2006) Comparison of two fluid-management strategies in acute lung injury. N Engl J Med 354:2564–2575
42. Dalfino L, Tullo L, Donadio I, et al. (2008) Intra-abdominal hipertensión and acute renal failure in critically ill patients. Intens Care Med 34:707–713
43. Malbrain ML, Cheatham ML, Kirkpatrick A, et al. (2006) Results from the international conference of experts on intra-abdominal hypertension and abdominal compartment syndrome. I. Definitions. Intens Care Med 32:1722–1732
44. Cheatham ML, Malbrain M, Kirkpatrick A, et al. (2007) Results from the international conference of experts on intra-abdominal hypertension and abdominal compartment syndrome. II. Recommendations. Intens Care Med 33:951–962
45. Garella S, Matarese RA (1984) Renal effects of prosta-glandins and clinical adverse effects of nonsteroidal antiinflammatory agents. Medicine 63:165–181
46. Barza M, Ioannidis JP, Cappelleri JC, Lau J (1996) Single or multiple daily doses of aminoglycosides: a meta-análisis. BMJ 312:338–344
47. Barrett BJ, Carlisle EJ (1993) Metaanalysis of the relative nephrotoxicity of high- and low-osmolality iodinated contrast media. Radiology 188:171–178
48. Solomon R, Deray G (2006) How to prevent contrast induced nephropathy and manage risk patients: practical recommendations. Proceedings of the contrast-induced nephropathy consensus panel. Kidney Int 69 (Suppl. 100):S51–S53
49. Venkataraman R, Kellum JA (2007) Prevention of acute renal failure. Chest 131:300–308
50. Holmes CL, Walley KR (2003) Low-dose dopamine in the ICU. Chest 123:1266–1275
51. Uchino S, Bellomo R, Morimatsu H, et al. (2007) Continuous renal replacement therapy: A worldwide practice survey. The beginning and ending supportive therapy for the kidney (BEST Kidney) investigators. Intens Care Med 33:1563–1570
52. Van Bommel EFH, Ponssen HH (1997) Intermittent versus continuous treatment for acute renal failure: Where do we stand? Am J Kidney Dis 30:S72–S79
53. Mehta RL (1997) Continuous renal replacement therapies in the acute renal failure setting: Current concepts. Adv Renal Replacement Ther 4:S81–S92

54. Bellomo R, Ronco C (1999) Continuous renal replacement therapy in the intensive care unit. Intens Care Med 25:781–789
55. Silvester W (1998) Outcome studies of continuous renal replacement therapy in the intensive care. Kidney Int 53:S138–S141
56. Mehta R, McDonald B, Gabbai F, et al. (1996) Continuous versus intermittent dialysis for acute renal failure in the ICU: results from a randomized multicenter trial. J Am Soc Nephrol 5:1457–1462
57. Kellum JA, Angus DC, Johnson JP, et al. (2002) Continuous versus intermittent renal replacement therapy: a meta-analysis. Intens Care Med 28: 29–37
58. Bell M, SWING, Granath F, Schön S, Ekbom A, Roland Martling C (2007) Continuous renal replacement therapy is associated with less chronic renal failure than intermittent haemodialysis alter acute renal failure. Intens Care Med 33:773–780
59. Bagshaw SM, Berthiaume LR, Delaney A, Bellomo R (2008) Continuous versus intermittent renal replacement therapy for critically ill patients with acute kidney injury: A meta-analysis. Crit Care Med 36:610–617
60. Chang JW, Yang WS, Seo JW, Lee JS, Lee SK, Park SK (2004) Continuous venovenous hemofiltration versus hemodiálisis as renal replacement therapy in patients with acute renal failure in the intensive care unit. Scand J Urol Nephrol 38:417–421
61. Vinsonneau Ch, Camus Ch, Combes A, et al. (Hemodiafe Study Group) (2006) Continuous venovenous haemofiltration versus intermittent haemodialysis for acute renal failure in patients with multiple-organ dysfunction síndrome: a randomised trial. Lancet 368:379–385
62. Uehlinger DE, Jakob SM, Ferrari P, et al. (2005) Comparison of continuous and intermittent renal replacement therapy for acute renal failure. Nephrol Dial Transplant 20:1630–1637
63. Augustine JJ, Sandy D, Seifert TH, Paganini EP (2004) A randomized controlled trial comparing intermittent with continuous dialysis in patients with ARF. Am J Kidney Dis 44: 1000–1007
64. Vanholder R, Van Biesen WIM, Lameire N (2001) What is the renal replacement method of first choice for intensive care patients? J Am Soc Nephrol 12:S40–S43
65. Ronco C, Bellomo R, Homel P, et al. (2000) Effects of different doses in continuous venovenous haemofiltration on outcomes of acute renal failure: a prospective randomised trial. Lancet 356:26–30
66. Schiffl H, Lang S, Fischer R (2002) Daily hemodialysis and the outcome of acute renal failure. N Eng J Med 346:305–310
67. The VA/NIH Acute Renal Failure Trial Network: Intensity of renal support in critically ill patients with acute kidney injury. N Engl J Med 2008 359:7–20
68. Several authors. (2008) Renal support in critically ill patients with acute kidney injury. N Engl J Med 359 (18):1959–1962
69. Honoré PM, Jamez J, Wauthier M, et al. (2000) Prospective evaluation of short-term, high-volume isovolemic hemofiltration on the hemodynamic course and outcome in patients with intractable circulatory failure resulting from septic shock. Crit Care Med 28:3581–3587
70. Jiang HL, Xue WJ, Li DQ, Yin AP, Xin X, Li CM, Gao JL (2005) Influence of continuous venovenous hemofiltration on the course of acute pancreatitis. World J Gastroenterol 11:4815–4821
71. Cole L, Bellomo R, Journois D, et al. (2001) High-volume haemofiltration in human septic shock. Intens Care Med 27:978–986
72. Luyckx VA and Bonventre JV (2004) Dose of dialysis in acute renal failure. Sem Dialysis 17:30–36
73. Maynar-Moliner J, Sánchez-Izquierdo-Riera JA, Herrera-Gutierrez M (2008) Renal support in critically ill patients with acute kidney injury. N Engl J Med 359:1960
74. Herrera Gutierrez M, Seller Pérez G, Lebrón Gallardo M, Muñoz Bono J, Banderas Bravo E, Cordón López A (2006) Early hemodynamic improvement is a prognostic marker in patients treated with continuous CVVHDF for acute renal failure. ASAIO J 52:670–676

75. Ricci Z, Ronco C, Bachetoni A, D'amico G, Rossi St (2006) Solute removal during continuous renal replacement therapy in critically ill patients: convection versus difusión. Crit Care 10:R67
76. Sander A, Armbruster W, Sander B, et al. (1995) The influence of continuous hemofiltration on cytokine elimination and the cardiovascular stability in the early phase of sepsis. Contrib Nephrol 116:99–103
77. Sanchez-Izquierdo Riera JA, Alted López E, Lozano Quintana MJ, et al. (1997) Influence of continuous hemofiltration on the hemodynamics of trauma patients. Surgery 122:902–908
78. Honoré PM, Joannes-Boyau O (2004) High volumen hemofiltration (HVHF) in sepsis: A comprehensive review of rationale, clinical applicability, potential indications and recommendations for future research. Int J Artif Org 27:1077–1082
79. Oudemans-Van Straaten HM, Bosman RJ, van der Spoel JI, Zandstra DF (1999) Outcome of critically ill patients treated with intermittent high-volume haemofiltration: a prospective cohort analysis. Intens Care Med 25:814–821
80. Joannes-Boyau O, Rapaport St, Bazin R, Fleureau C, Janvier G (2004) Impact of high volume hemofiltration on hemodynamic disturbance and outcome during septic shock. ASAIO J 50:102–109
81. Ratanarat R, Brendolan A, Piccinni P, et al. (2005) Pulse high-volume haemofiltration for treatment of severe sepsis: effects on hemodynamics and survival. Crit Care 9:R294–R302
82. Piccinni P, Dan M, Barbacini St, et al. (2006) Early isovolemic haemofiltration in oliguric patients with septic shock. Intens Care Med 32:80–86
83. Hoffman JN, Hartl WH, Deppisch, et al. (1995) Hemofiltration in human sepsis: evidence for elimination of immunomodulatory substances. Kidney Int 48:1563–1570
84. Braun N, Rosenfeld S, Giolai M, et al. (1995) Effects of continuous hemodiafiltration on IL-6, TNF-alfa, C3a, and TCC in patients with SIRS/septic shock using two different membranes. Contrib Nephrol 116:89–98
85. Ronco C, Tetta C, Lupi A, et al. (1995) Removal of platelet-activating factor in experimental continuous arteriovenous hemofiltration. Crit Care Med 23:99–107
86. Heering P, Morgera S, Schmitz FJ, et al. (1997) Cytokine removal and cardiovascular hemodynamics in septic patients with continuous veno-venous hemofiltration. Intens Care Med 23:288–296
87. Ronco C, Tetta C, Mariano F, et al. (2003) Interpreting the mechanisms of continuous renal replacement therapy in sepsis: the peak concentration hypothesis. Artif Organs 27:792–801
88. Yekebas EF, Eisenberger C, Ohnesorge H, Saalmuller A, Elsner H, Engelhart M, et al. (2001) Attenuation of sepsis-related immunoparalysis by continuous veno-venous hemofiltration in experimental porcine pancreatitis. Crit Care Med 29:1423–1430
89. Sanchez-Izquierdo Riera JA, Pérez Vela JL, Lozano Quintana MJ, et al. (1997) Cytokines clearance during venovenous hemofiltration in the trauma patient. Am J Kidney Dis 30:483–488
90. Haase M, Bellomo R, Baldwin I, et al. (2007) Hemodialysis membrane with a high-molecular-weight cutoff and cytokine levels in sepsis complicated by acute renal failure: A Phase 1 randomized trial. Am J Kidney Dis 50:296–304
91. Fortin MC, Amyot SL, Geadah D, Leblanc M (1999) Serum concentrations and clearances of folic acid and pyridoxal-5′-phosphate during venovenous continuous renal replacement therapy. Crit Care Med 25:594–598
92. Story DA, Ronco C, Bellomo R (1999) Trace element and vitamin concentrations and losses in critically ill patients treated with continuous venovenous hemofiltration. Crit Care Med 27:220–223
93. Berger MM, Shenkin A, Revelly JP, et al. (2004) Copper, selenium, zinc, and thiamine balances during continuous venovenous hemodiafiltration in critically ill patients. Am J Clin Nutr 80:410–416
94. Maynar J (2007) Extracoporeal clearance and extracorporeal clearance fraction: pharmacokinetic bases and drug dosing in continuous extracorporeal treatments. Nefrologia 27(3):247–255
95. Moran SM, Myers BD (1985) Course of acute renal failure studied by a model of creatinine kinetics. Kidney Int 27:928–927

Immunoglobulin, Sepsis, and Pneumonia

Jordi Almirall, Ester Vendrell, and Javier de Gracia

1
The Pathogenesis of Infection

Infectious disease is defined as a set of signs and symptoms that result from inflammation or dysfunction of one or more organs caused by a microorganism or its components. This can be due to infection, if the etiological agent multiplies in the host, or intoxication if it is due to the toxins generated by a microorganism.

In the pathogenesis of the infection, the components of the microorganisms that induce the inflammatory response and the defense mechanisms of the host must be considered. The balance between the microbial virulence and the immunity of the host determines the final result of the process, the magnitude and nature of the triggered inflammatory response conditioning the signs and symptoms, gravity, and course of the disease.

The defense mechanisms of the host include:

1. The cutaneous–mucous barrier. The morphological integrity of the skin and mucous membranes provides an effective primary defense barrier. Invasion of microorga-nisms must be preceded by physical/chemical mechanisms modifying this barrier. Epithelial surfaces have mechanical, chemical, and microbiological barriers against infection. Normal flora compete with pathogens for binding sites and essential nutrients and also produce inhibiting substances.
2. *Innate Immunity.* Recognition of molecular patterns of pathogens allows the differentiation of a series of microbial components detailed below.

Humoral immunity is formed by antimicrobial peptides, complement, and coagulation. Anti-microbial peptides are present in the whole range of multicellular organisms and have the specific function of collaborating with other components of innate immunity

J. Almirall (✉)
Critical Care Unit, Hospital de Mataró, Universitat Autònoma de Barcelona, Ciber Enfermedades Respiratorias (CibeRes), Barcelona
e-mail: jalmirall@csdm.cat

in order to neutralize or delay the dissemination of the pathogens while the adaptive response is being organized. Complement was originally identified as a thermolabile serum that "complemented" the antibodies in bacteria lysis. It comprises a group of over 30 serum proteins that interact in a coordinated way, forming the complement cascade. This can be activated by specific antibodies or by molecules, particularly extracellular, found on the surface of the microorganisms. More recently, a third way has been described: activation by microbial carbohydrates.

Cellular immunity occurs through a phagocytosis process, the cells most implicated being: polymorphonuclear leukocytes (neutrophils, basophils, and eosinophils); macrophages (that develop from monocytes), which are important producers of proinflammatory cytokines, mainly, interleukin (IL)-1, tumor necrosis factor (TNF)-alpha, IL-12, IL-10, and IL-8; mast cells that are activated when pathogens cross the epithelial barrier and establish a local infection; dendritic cells that act between innate and adaptive immunities; and finally "natural killer" cells, which are an important source of interferon gamma in the innate immune response to cell production.

3. *Adaptive Immunity* occurs when the innate system is overloaded and involves the participation of cellular and humoral mechanisms that act specifically against the infectious agents, generating an immunological memory. This process is mediated by antigens presented by antigen-presenting cells activating B and T lymphocytes that produce plasma cells which in turn produce antibodies. Antibodies are complex glycoproteins that bind to the microbial antigens, activating microbicide reactions. They are formed by a variable region where they bind to the antigen and a constant region responsible for initiating the activation of the complement, the antibody-dependent cellular cytotoxicity or phagocytosis. The constant regions of the antibodies determine the five classes of immunoglobulins: IgM, IgG, IgA, IgD, and IgE. Classes IgG and IgA are divided into subclasses according to the different genes that encode their corresponding heavy chains. In the case of respiratory infection, the microorganism that invades the lung provokes a defensive mechanism which includes immunoglobulins, especially IgA, IgM, IgG, and their subclasses. These immunoglobulins reach the respiratory tract by diffusion from the blood or by in situ production in the existing lymphoid tissue in the respiratory tract. The main function of immunoglobulins in the lung is to inhibit attachment of the pathogens to the respiratory epithelium and to facilitate their destruction by phagocyte cells.

IgA is the immunoglobulin with the greatest in situ production. Almost all IgA found in the respiratory tract is of local production and is dimeric, while in serum it is monomeric. Its main function is to neutralize inhaled antigens through an agglutination mechanism that allows the immunoglobulin to bind with the bacteria, thus preventing them from attaching and colonizing in the respiratory epithelium.

Under normal conditions, only small quantities of IgM are found in the respiratory tract.

IgG is the predominant immunoglobulin in the lower respiratory tract. The proportion of IgG subclasses is similar to that in serum, except for IgG2 which is greater in nonsmokers [1]. There are four subclasses, with the main ones being IgG3 and IgG4 [2].

Any defect in immunoglobulin synthesis, and particularly IgG, could favor respiratory infection and the presence of colonized pathogens in the respiratory tract. This has been demonstrated in recurrent respiratory infections.

2
Community-Acquired Pneumonia: An Old Challenge

2.1
Morbidity and Mortality

Pneumonia is a prevalent cause of sepsis and a potentially life-threatening condition, yet most patients do not need hospitalization and can be cured without sequelae. Data from European studies estimate the prevalence of community-acquired pneumonia (CAP) at 2–10 cases per 1,000 of the general adult population per year, this number increasing to 25–35 cases when considering patients older than 70 years [3]. The frequency of the condition is age related, with the highest rates in the very young and very old [4].

Both community-acquired and nosocomial pneumonia contribute substantially to morbidity, the need for hospitalization being estimated at 35% of patients [3], which represents an important burden to the healthcare system. In some U.S. studies, CAP alone causes over one million hospital admissions annually and $4.4 billion in hospitalization costs [5].

The overall estimated mortality attributable to CAP is five million deaths per year in the world. It is the sixth most common cause of death and the main cause of death from infection in industrialized countries [3, 6]. Mortality varies according to the causative agent and individual risk factors, ranging from 2 to 53% in some studies [7].

Bacteremia is known to be related to a worse CAP prognosis, but positive blood cultures are not obtained immediately and initial decisions must be taken without this information. Moreover, blood cultures are only positive in 1–16% of patients hospitalized with CAP [6], and their negativity does not exclude sepsis.

The more hemodynamically affected patients are, the less chance they have of surviving, following the physiopathology of sepsis [7, 8]. Thus, clinical and laboratory features at presentation need continuous surveillance over the first hours or days, in the acute phase of CAP, in order to detect any sign that would indicate the need for a change in therapeutic decisions [9, 10]. Initial management is, therefore, very important. Guide-lines should be available in emergency departments where the use of severity scores to assess and predict patient outcome can be useful in detecting patients in need of more intensive treatment.

Severity scores used to help make first-line medical decisions are continuously being evaluated [8, 11]. The Pneumonia Severity Index (PSI) and CURB-65 predict mortality well but are less appropriate for taking site-of-care decisions, whereas the revised American Thoracic Society score (rATS) seems to identify the need for ICU admission well, but does not help predict mortality. Severity score validation must be undertaken according to the clinical context because sensitivity and specificity can vary. It is important for clinicians to know what they can expect from each tool.

Because of the clinical and economic impact of pneumonia, it is important to identify and fully understand all modifiable factors that influence its natural course [5]. Several epidemiological and clinical studies have been conducted to detect specific predisposing factors to lower tract infection [6]. Recurrent pneumonia is associated with defects in host defenses, including leukocyte function and immunoglobulin production in children and young adults. Other important predisposing conditions in younger and older populations are structural lung abnormalities such as bronchiectasis and pulmonary sequestration. Congenital defects in each stage of the respiratory defense system would also predispose children and young adults to recurrent infections of the respiratory tract [12–16]. In this case the clinician must be ready to investigate potential underlying immunologic abnormalities in order to take the corresponding preventive or therapeutic measures: polysaccharide antigen vaccines and substitutive immunoglobulin treatment [17–22].

2.2
Immunoglobulins and Capsular Polysaccharides

The most frequently found pathogens in bronchial secretions of respiratory infections are capsular Gram-positive bacteria, *Streptococcus pneumoniae* being the most prevalent [3]. In the laboratory, these pathogens are identified and subdivided according to their capsular antigen into different strains and serotypes [23]. The specific protective immunoglobulins recognize these capsular antigens following the physiopathology of adaptive immunity detailed above.

The most immunogenic bacterial antigens are the peripheral ones: capsular proteins and lipopolysaccharide, among others. These peripheral antigen proteins have been used in clinical practice as vaccines to deliberately trigger a specific immune response against these pathogens [23].

The capsular antigens are purified of selected pathogens to induce the production of specific immunoglobulins. With regard to CAP, *S. pneumoniae* (19.3%) is the causal organism most frequently isolated, followed by *Haemophilus influenza* (3.3%) [3, 4]. Although the etiologic agent is not identified in 49.8% of cases, the preventive strategies must be directed towards guaranteeing immunological protection against these two pathogens that are present temporarily or permanently in normal flora in the respiratory tract in a high percentage of the population.

All this helps explain the physiopathology of sepsis in pneumonia. As with all kinds of sepsis, the immunological cascade is activated and although there is not much scientific evidence available, we suggest that there is a hypothetical consumption of specific immunoglobulins in patients with lung infections. For example, in our study of 181 adult CAP patients, in the acute phase we observed a significant decrease in IgA, IgG in general, and some specific subclasses of IgG, particularly IgG2 (Table 1) [24]. Other authors have also studied the changes in Ig serum concentrations in the acute phase and convalescence of pneumonia, but there is insufficient consistency between the studies as the conditions under which they were performed vary markedly [25–27]. Some studies have detected a further decrease in IgG subclasses in patients with known deficiency [28]. Others have followed the levels of immunoglobulins from diagnosis to the acute phase of CAP and convalescence, where most find a normalization of levels (Tables 2 and 3) [24, 25, 27], while other authors have not detected changes [26] or not obtained enough follow-up data to come to reliable conclusions [7].

Table 1 Mean concentrations of Ig (mg dL^{-1}) in acute-phase CAP

	IgG_1	IgG_2	IgG_3	IgG_4	IgG_{TOTAL}	IgA	IgM
CAP cases	521	240	44.5	31	820	200	110
Controls	651	328.5	52.5	38	1120	245	100
p	<0.001	<0.001	0.05	0.3	<0.001	<0.001	0.2

From Almirall et al. [24]
CAP community-acquired pneumonia

Table 2 Changes in percentage of patients with and without immunoglobulin deficiency from clinical diagnosis of CAP to convalescence at 30 days

	Immunological state on clinical diagnosis	Immunological state at convalescence
	Initial cases with follow-up: n (%)	Final cases with follow-up: n (%)
Total number of cases	110 (100%)	110 (100%)
– With normal Igs	57 (51.8%)	83 (75.5%)
– With deficient levels of Igs	53 (48.2%)	27 (24.5%)
• Hypogammaglobulinemia	15	5
• ↓IgG total	38[a]	20[b]
• ↓IgG2	29[a]	15[a]
• Other Igs	2	1

From Almirall et al. [24]
Ig immunoglobulin, *CAP* community-acquired pneumonia
[a] Sixteen of these patients also had low levels of total IgG and IgG2
[b] Nine of these patients also had low levels of total IgG and IgG2

2.2.1
Adaptive Immunity: Induction and Impairment

Impairments at every stage of the pulmonary defense system can predispose to infections, and each stage can be affected by a number of factors. For example, alcohol and cigarette smoke can impair mucociliary function, macrophage activity, and other immunologic responses in the lung [6, 21]. Other external noxa are known to interfere with normal ciliary function, such as, *Mycoplasma pneumoniae, H. influenzae*, and viruses. Some of the latter may also inhibit alveolar macrophage or neutrophil function [6], and *Chlamydia* are said to affect mucociliary clearance in COPD patients [29]. Intrinsic structural lung abnormalities such as bronchiectasis, tuberculous cavernomas, or emphysematous bullae also predispose to infection of the lung secretions, as demonstrated in COPD patients.

Table 3 Immunoglobulin progression

	IgG$_2$				IgG				IgG or any IgG subclass			
	N–N	L–N	L–L	p	N–N	L–N	L–L	p	N–N	L–N	L–L	p
Sex												
Male (n = 66)	69	20	10		59	21	20		48	26	26	
Female (n = 82)	80	9	11	0.3	75	14	11	0.3	57	20	23	0.7
Repeated respiratory infection												
Yes (n = 15)	80	8	12		72	12	16		64	8	28	
No (n = 82)	73	18	9	0.4	63	21	16	0.6	49	29	22	0.07
Chronic bronchitis												
Yes (n = 26)	77	15	8		61	23	15		50	31	19	
No (n = 18)	74	16	10	1.0	67	17	16	0.8	53	22	25	0.7
History of CAP												
Yes (n = 17)	88	6	6		71	23	6		65	23	12	
No (n = 89)	72	18	10	0.5	64	18	18	0.5	50	24	25	0.5
CAP severity												
Treated at home (n = 52)	74	12	14		75	11	13		54	21	25	
Hospitalized (n = 58)	72	19	9	0.4	57	24	19	0.1	50	26	24	0.8
Microbiology												
Not studied (n = 60)	71	12	17		57	23	20		45	27	28	
Bacteria (n = 33)	76	21	3		70	12	18		55	21	24	
Virus (n = 12)	67	25	8		83	17	0		58	25	17	
Bacteria and virus (n = 5)	100	0	0	0.3	100	0	0	0.3	100	0	0	0.5
Caused by Pneumococcus												
Yes (n = 19)	100	25	8		89	5	5		84	5	10	
No (n = 91)	67	0	0	0.01	60	21	19	0.08	45	27	27	.009
Caused by Chlamydia												
Yes (n = 8)	62	37	0		62	37	0		37	62	0	
No (n = 102)	74	14	12	0.2	66	17	18	0.2	53	21	26	0.02

Comparison of percentage of patients with normal or low immunological levels from clinical diagnosis of CAP to convalescence at 30 days
From Almirall et al. [24]
IgG total immunoglobulin G; *IgG$_2$* immunoglobulin IgG subclass 2; *N–N* percentage of patients with normal levels initially and at the convalescent phase; *L–N* percentage of patients having normalized their initial low levels; *L–L* percentage of patients with persistently low levels

The challenge, however, is to cure the infection at the focus itself, where the opsonized proteins play the main role. In fact, immunoglobulins, which have been studied for over 20 years, are the key, the link between the lung defense systems and the respiratory pathogens.

Subnormal levels of one or several IgG subclasses may be relatively common, and certain subclass deficiencies may not be clinically relevant and thus it is important to define the normal range, not always measured in the same way in the literature [13]. Moreover, deficient immunoglobulin production does not affect mortality rates [7], but nevertheless, the predisposition of patients with immunoglobulin deficiency, complete or incomplete, isolated or combined, to suffer from repeated bronchial infections with consequent bronchiectasis or recurrent CAP has been studied by several authors [7, 12, 13, 15, 17, 22, 30–32].

2.2.2
Response to Immunization

All the issues mentioned thus far lead to the recommendation to vaccinate patients most at risk from recurrent bronchial infections with the capsular polysaccharides of the respiratory pathogens. However, deficient immunoglobulin production does not only result in a certain defenselessness of the patient against the capsular pathogen but also a weaker vaccinal response [22, 33–35]. Some studies have found partial responses, but they reach plasma levels not always considered sufficient to guarantee adequate immunological protection [17, 26, 34, 36]. Some authors have proposed the theory that IgG2 is a more specific immunoglobulin against pneumococcal polysaccharides, leading to a subclass-specific inducing or regulating mechanism for human response to polysaccharide antigens [14, 37]. This would explain the fact that in some cases a diminished IgG2 has been detected in the acute phase of pneumonia [24, 27].

Several authors have studied a booster effect of a second dose of immunization. In the case of pneumococci, for example, the specific immunoglobulin reached protective levels on the administration of a second vaccine (polyvalent polysaccharide) 6 months after having a partial or null response to the first vaccine (conjugated) [36]. This effect after a second attempt at immunization has not always been confirmed, however, probably due to immune diversity in which the immunoglobulin deficits could be transitory, particularly in children [38].

Again an adequate response to pneumococcal immunization needs further definition. It is clear, however, that age has an important influence on the intensity of the response to most pneumococcal polysaccharides, which means that studies need to be read carefully in order to avoid misinterpretation of the data [39].

2.3
Immunoglobulins and Their Subclasses

As mentioned above, the immunoglobulins that act mainly in the lung are the subclasses of IgG, in particular IgG2, IgG3, and IgG4 [20].

Studies on IgG subclasses have been performed since the 1960s, when patients with repeated bronchial infections, especially those caused by capsular bacteria, were detected as having some IgG subclass deficiency. Some studies detected over 10% of patients with some impairment in immunoglobulin levels [13, 20]. The differentiation of congenital from acquired deficiencies dates to 1990.

Each subclass can be deficient in an isolated or combined way and thus each deficiency can predispose to different kinds of infections [14]. However, there is scarce literature on immunoglobulins in adult patients with recurrent infections.

In primary immunodeficiencies, the selective deficiency of IgA is the most prevalent [17], but IgG2 deficiency, associated or not with IgA and/or IgG4, has been the most closely associated with an increased incidence of recurrent respiratory infections, especially in children and youths [12, 34] and also patients with CAP [35, 40]. Selective deficiency of IgG3 or IgG4 as risk factors for recurrent respiratory infections is disputed and when an association is found, other immunological impairments or concomitant risk factors must be discounted. This is also the case with IgG4 deficiency, which is associated with recurrent and severe pulmonary infections and is therefore closely related to bronchiectasis [20, 31, 32].

Nonprimary deficiencies, especially IgG and IgG2, can be secondary to other pathologies such as thymoma, lymphoproliferative disorders, malabsorption, intestinal surgery, and alcoholic liver disease among others [13, 20, 21] with similar consequences to those of primary deficiencies.

Some studies, including one by this author, aim to detect patients at risk of having an immunoglobulin deficiency to give some kind of applicable solution in clinical practice, as explained below [7, 26, 41, 29].

3
Immunoglobulins in Clinical Practice

As mentioned, there can be several potential impairments in the specific immune response in the lung, but the most well-known and most studied is congenital deficiency of immunoglobulins. If such abnormalities are detected, preventive measures must be taken, i.e., capsulated vaccines or immune treatment.

There is a large amount of evidence that parenteral substitutive treatment with the defective specific immunoglobulin, or else with a combination of immunoglobulins, can at least minimize recurrent bronchial infections and postpone lung destruction from consequent bronchiectasis and recurrent episodes, breaking the vicious circle [12–16, 20, 42, 43]. More data are needed to ascertain whether this beneficial effect is linked to a reduction in infection-related morbidity and mortality [44]. However, its effectiveness in reducing serious infections is so evident that proposing double-blind studies is not considered ethical.

In some cases the immunological deficiency is less evident. For example, normal levels of immunoglobulins can be found in cases of repeated respiratory infection. In these cases, subclasses of IgG should be examined [45, 46]. Likewise, immunoglobulins and their subclasses may have normal levels but the physiological response may be deficient. By vaccinating the patients with capsular polysaccharides, an impaired IgG antibody response to polysaccharide antigens will be evident, whereas normal serum titers of IgG antibodies will be obtained in respose to the innoculation of other antigenic proteins, such as tetanus toxoid [20, 22, 30].

Subsequently, before indicating immunoglobulin treatment, a detailed study should be done to investigate specific immune response to vaccines [22]. In some situations, such as non-responsiveness to polysaccharide vaccine, the possibility of a generalized nonresponsiveness to polysaccharide antigens can be considered; these patients would be contenders for periodic administration of parenteral immunoglobulins [17].

However, there is still insufficient scientific evidence for the use of parenteral immunoglobulins as therapy in acute-phase CAP. In response to the apparent consumption of immunoglobulins, particularly IgG2 in the acute phase of CAP [27], studies have been undertaken to assess the possible benefits of its administration to patients with a specific subclass deficiency [12, 17, 19, 22, 42]. However, these are isolated studies, not easily comparable, and this treatment has not been included in clinical practice yet.

As shown above, intravenous immunoglobulin prophylaxis can undoubtedly reduce the occurrence of pneumonias in at-risk patients [44]; moreover, more and more studies are recommending the administration of this immune protein in the acute phase of lung infection [10, 14–16, 18, 20, 21, 47, 48] because of the physiopathology of lung destruction in CAP. The exogenous immunoglobulins supplement the deficient local function in affected patients, avoiding the detrimental side effects of the whole immune cascade that would be triggered by other molecules (complements, etc.).

So far we have discussed lung infections, and in particular their relationship with the dysfunction of certain subclasses of IgG2. We will now discuss the implication of immunoglobulin deficiency on sepsis in general. We can state that death from severe sepsis and septic shock is common, and studies have explored whether antibodies to the endotoxins in some bacteria reduce mortality [49, 50]. Studies on laboratory animals show significantly improved survival and pulmonary histopathology by the administration of high-dose intravenous immunoglobulin (1,000 mg kg^{-1}) [51]. A meta-analysis has also been undertaken on randomized controlled trials including adult and child patients, which has confirmed the significant effect of immunoglobulin treatment on mortality in sepsis and septic shock [52].

The use of intravenous immunoglobulin in severe sepsis and septic shock in adults does not replace the standard treatment of antibiotics and corticosteroids among other medications; however, the initial choice of antibiotic continues to have a dramatic effect on outcome [9, 10, 44]. Regarding the type of immunoglobulin used, polyvalent immunoglobulin seems more effective in several studies. A reduction in mortality by pooled intravenous IgG enriched with IgA and IgM more than by intravenous IgG alone was reported in the recent Cochrane database (eight trials, 492 patients) [44] and similar results were found in another meta-analysis that selected adults and neonates with sepsis [52].

However, significant heterogeneity exists among the majority of these trials and further investigation is needed [50].

The most recent UK Department of Health guidelines on prescribing intravenous immunoglobulin, and the American Society of Health-System Pharmacists' indications, both published in 2008, describe similar recommendations to give priority to patients according to the risk of no treatment [10, 53]. The labeled indications in immunology are impaired specific antibody production, Kawasaki disease, and primary immunodeficiencies among others, whereas a low priority is given to secondary antibody deficiencies because of weak evidence. If we focus on infectious diseases, intravenous immunoglobulin use would be priority in toxic shock syndrome, necrotizing staphylococcal sepsis, severe invasive group A streptococcal disease, severe or recurrent *Clostridium difficile* colitis, and viral infections such as general parvovirus infection, rotaviral enterocolitis, respiratory syncytial virus, lower respiratory tract infection, and Cytomegalovirus infection in solid organ transplant. The treatment is not recommended for sepsis in the ICU not related to specific toxins or *C. difficile* [54].

Finally, there are differences between the guidelines. During neonatal sepsis or in pediatric patients with immunodeficiency secondary to HIV infection, intravenous immunoglobulin treatment is not recommended in the UK guidelines, whereas this condition does have some evidence-based indication for the American pharmacists. The 2008 international guidelines for management of severe sepsis give support to the use of polyclonal intravenous immunoglobulin in pediatric population, since it has been shown to have favorable outcomes such as less mortality and less progress to complications with an evidence grade 2C [56].

Intravenous immunoglobulin also has an unlabeled indication in patients with immunosuppression due to IgG subclass deficiency with severe infection, as well as in bone marrow transplant to prevent infections [53].

To sum up, in any chronic, recurrent, or unusual infections, not only recurrent bronchial infections, diagnosis of immune deficiency should be considered. For patients who lack immunoglobulins and antibodies, intravenous immunoglobulin, given monthly and continued throughout life, is the standard of care [56]. On the other hand, in the treatment of sepsis and septic shock, intravenous immunoglobulins are already being used as prophylaxis and as supplementary treatment in sepsis [44]. Future and ongoing studies will document further benefit from intravenous immunoglobulin treatment in different septic processes [44, 50, 57, 58].

References

1. Reynolds HY (1987) Host defense impairments that may lead to respiratory infections. Clin Chest Med 8(3):339–358
2. Holland SM, Gallin JI (2005) Evaluation of the patient with suspected immunodeficiency. In: Mandell GL, Bennett JE, Dolin (eds) Principles and practice of infectious diseases, 6th ed. Elsevier, Philadelphia, pp. 2–3
3. Almirall J, Bolibar I, Vidal J, Sauca G, Coll P, Niklasson B, Bartolomé M, Balanzó X (2000) Epidemiology of community-acquired pneumonia in adults: a population-based study. Eur Respir J 15:757–763
4. Woodhead M (2002) Community-acquired pneumonia in Europe: causative pathogens and resistance patterns. Eur Respir J(Suppl 36):20s–27s
5. Zilberberg MD, Exuzides A, Spalding J, Foreman A, Jones AG, Colby C, Shorr AF (2008) Hyponatremia and hospital outcomes among patients with pneumonia: a retrospective cohort study. BMC Pulm Med 18(8):16
6. Donowitz GR, Mandell GL (2005) Acute pneumonia. In: Mandell GL, Bennett JE, Dolin (eds) Principles and practice of infectious diseases, 6th ed. Elsevier, Philadelphia
7. Feldman C, Mahomed AG, Mahida P, Morar R, Schoeman A, Mpe J, Burgin S, Kuschke RH, Wadee A (1996) IgG subclasses in previously healthy adult patients with acute community-acquired pneumonia. S Afr Med J 86(5 Suppl):600–602

8. Valencia M, Badia JR, Cavalcanti M, Ferrer M, Agustí C, Angrill J, García E, Mensa J, Niederman MS, Torres A (2007) Pneumonia severity index class v patients with community-acquired pneumonia: characteristics, outcomes, and value of severity scores. Chest 132(2):515–522
9. Bautista MD, Bravo-Rodríguez F, Fuentes F, Sancho H (2004) Glucocorticoids and immunoglobulins in an acute respiratory distress syndrome secondary to varicella pneumoniae. Med Clin 122:238–238
10. Rodríguez A, Rello J, Neira J, Maskin B, Ceraso D, Vasta L, Palizas F (2005) Effects of high-dose of intravenous immunoglobulin and antibiotics on survival for severe sepsis undergoing surgery. Shock 23(4):298–304
11. Buising KL, Thursky KA, Black JF, MacGregor L, Street AC, Kennedy MP, Brown GV (2006) A prospective comparison of severity scores for identifying patients with severe community acquired pneumonia: reconsidering what is meant by severe pneumonia. Thorax 61(5):419–424
12. Ekdahl K, Braconier JH, Rollof J (1992) Recurrent pneumonia: a review of 90 adult patients. Scand J Infect Dis 24(1):71–76
13. Hanson LA, Söderström R, Avanzini A, Bengtsson U, Björkander J, Söderström T (1988) Immunoglobulin subclass deficiency. Pediatr Infect Dis J 7(5 Suppl):S17–S21
14. Jefferis R, Kumararatne DS (1990) Selective IgG subclass deficiency: quantification and clinical relevance. Clin Exp Immunol 81(3):357–367
15. Martínez MA, Hernández FD (2000) Inmunodeficiencias primarias y afectación pulmonar. Reuniones anuales: ponencias de la edición de 2004. Primera ponencia, parte II: infecciones y función pulmonar. http://www.alergoaragon.org/2004/primera3.html
16. Shield JP, Strobel S, Levinsky RJ, Morgan G (1992) Immunodeficiency presenting as hypergammaglobulinaemia with IgG2 subclass deficiency. Lancet 340(8817):448–450
17. Ekdahl K, Braconier JH, Svanborg C (1997) Immunoglobulin deficiencies and impaired immune response to polysaccharide antigens in adult patients with recurrent community-acquired pneumonia. Scand J Infect Dis 29(4):401–407
18. Heiner DC (1986) IgG subclass composition of intravenous immunoglobulin preparations: clinical relevance. Rev Infect Dis 8(Suppl 4):S391–S395
19. Knutsen AP (1989) Patients with IgG subclass and/or selective antibody deficiency to polysaccharide antigens: initiation of a controlled clinical trial of intravenous immune globulin. J Allergy Clin Immunol 84:640–647
20. Morell A (1994) Clinical relevance of IgG subclass deficiencies. Ann Biol Clin (Paris) 52(1):49–52
21. Spinozzi F, Cimignoli E, Gerli R, Agea E, Bertotto A, Rondoni F, Grignani F (1992) IgG subclass deficiency and sinopulmonary bacterial infections in patients with alcoholic liver disease. Arch Int Med 152(1):99–104
22. Vendrell M, de Gracia J, Rodrigo MJ, Cruz MJ, Alvarez A, Garcia M, Miravitlles M (2005) Antibody production deficiency with normal IgG levels in bronchiectasis of unknown etiology. Chest 127(1):197–204
23. Ausina V, Prats G (2006) Principales grupos de seres vivos con capacidad patógena para el hombre. In: Ausina V, Moreno S (ed) Tratado SEIMC de enfermedades infecciosas y microbiología clínica. Editorial Médica Panamericana, Madrid
24. Almirall J, de Gracia J (1993–1995) Internal register, Intensive Care Unit. Hospital de Mataró, Barcelona
25. Francoz D, Lapointe JM, Wellemans V, Desrochers A, Caswell JL, Stott JL, Dubreuil P (2004) Immunoglobulin G2 deficiency with transient hypogammaglobulinemia and chronic respiratory disease in a 6-month-old Holstein heifer. J Vet Diagn Invest 16(5):432–435
26. Herer B, Labrousse F, Mordelet-Dambrine M, Durandy A, Offredo-Hemmer C, Ekindjian O, Chretien J, Huchon G (1990) Selective IgG subclass deficiencies and antibody responses to pneumococcal capsular polysaccharide antigen in adult community-acquired pneumonia. Am Rev Respir Dis 142(4):854–857

27. Hukuhara H, Shigeno Y, Saito A (1991) Serum levels of healthy adult humans and changes of IgG subclass levels between infected and convalescent phase in respiratory infections. Kansenshogaku Zasshi 65(5):564–570
28. Söderström T, Söderström R, Andersson R, Lindberg J, Hanson LA (1988) Factors influencing IgG subclass levels in serum and mucosal secretions. Monogr Allergy 23:236–243
29. Blasi F, Aliberti S, Allegra L, Piatti G, Tarsia P, Ossewaarde JM, Verweij V, Nijkamp FP, Folkerts G (2007) Chlamydophila pneumoniae induces a sustained airway hyperresponsiveness and inflammation in mice. Respir Res 19(8):83
30. Bokszczanin A, Levinson AI (2003) Coexistent yellow nail syndrome and selective antibody deficiency. Ann Allergy Asthma Immunol 91(5):496–500
31. de José Gomez MI, González de Dios J, Hernando de Larramendi C, Jiménez García A, Vidal López ML, García Hortelano J (1990) IgG2 deficiency associated with recurrent pneumonia and asthma (review of an IgG subclass). An Esp Pediatr 33(3):258–264
32. Ninomiya H, Hasegawa H, Fukuoka T, Shiosaka T, Yamauchi T, Saiki O, Fujita S, Kobayashi Y (1991) Selective IgG2,4 subclass and IgE deficiencies in an adult patient with recurrent pneumonia. Jpn J Med 30(4):339–342
33. Dhooge IJ, van Kempen MJ, Sanders LA, Rijkers GT (2002) Deficient IgA and IgG2 antipneumococcal antibody levels and response to vaccination in otitis prone children. Int J Pediatr Otorhinolaryngol 17; 64(2):133–141
34. Sorensen RU, Hidalgo H, Moore C, Leiva LE (1996) Post-immunization pneumococcal antibody titers and IgG subclasses. Pediatr Pulmonol 22(3):167–173
35. Van Kessel DA, Horikx PE, Van Houte AJ, De Graaff CS, Van Velzen-Blad H, Rijkers GT (1999) Clinical and immunological evaluation of patients with mild IgG1 deficiency. Clin Exp Immunol 118(1):102–107
36. Breukels MA, Rijkers GT, Voorhorst-Ogink MM, Zegers BJ, Sanders LA (1999) Pneumococcal conjugate vaccine primes for polysaccharide-inducible IgG2 antibody response in children with recurrent otitis media acuta. J Infect Dis 179(5):1152–1156
37. Barrett DJ, Ayoub EM (1986) IgG2 subclass restriction of antibody to pneumococcal polysaccharides. Clin Exp Immunol 63(1):127–134
38. Sanders LA, Rijkers GT, Kuis W, Tenbergen-Meekes AJ, de Graeff-Meeder BR, Hiemstra I, Zegers BJ (1993) Defective antipneumococcal polysaccharide antibody response in children with recurrent respiratory tract infections. J Allergy Clin Immunol 91(1 Pt 1):110–119
39. Sorensen RU, Leiva LE, Javier FC 3rd, Sacerdote DM, Bradford N, Butler B, Giangrosso PA, Moore C (1998) Influence of age on the response to *Streptococcus pneumoniae* vaccine in patients with recurrent infections and normal immunoglobulin concentrations. J Allergy Clin Immunol 102(2):215–221
40. Miravitlles M, de Gracia J, Rodrigo MJ, Cruz MJ, Vendrell M, Vidal R, Morell F (1999) Specific antibody response against the 23-valent pneumococcal vaccine in patients with alpha(1)-antitrypsin deficiency with and without bronchiectasis. Chest 116(4):946–952
41. Beard LJ, Ferrante A, Oxelius VA, Maxwell GM (1986) IgG subclass deficiency in children with IgA deficiency presenting with recurrent or severe respiratory infections. Pediatr Res 20(10):937–942
42. Björkander J, Bake B, Oxelius VA, Hanson LA (1985) Impaired lung function in patients with IgA deficiency and low levels of IgG2 or IgG3. N Engl J Med 313:720–724
43. De Gracia J, Vendrell M, Álvarez A, Pallisa E, Rodrigo M-J, De la Rosa D, Mata F, Andreu J, Morell F (2004) Immunoglobulin therapy to control lung damage in patients with common variable immunodeficiency. Int Immunopharmacol 6:745–753
44. Werdan K (2001) Intravenous immunoglobulin for prophylaxis and therapy of sepsis. Curr Opin Crit Care 7(5):354–361
45. Loh RK, Harth SC, Thong YH, Ferrante A (1990) Immunoglobulin G subclass deficiency and predisposition to infection in Down's syndrome. Pediatr Infect Dis J 9(8):547–551

46. Wood P (2007) Recognition, clinical diagnosis and management of patients with primary antibody deficiencies: a systematic review. Clin Exp Immunol Sep:149(3):410–423. Epub 2007 Jun 12. Review
47. Chetan G, Mahadevan S, Sulanthung K, Narayanan P (2007) Intravenous immunoglobulin therapy of lupus pneumonitis. Indian J Pediatr 74(11):1032–1033
48. Sakiyama Y, Komiyama A, Shiraki K, Taniguchi N, Torii S, Baba S, Yata J, Matsumoto S (1998) Intravenous immunoglobulin (GB-0998) for prophylaxis of recurrent acute otitis media and lower respiratory tract infection in infancy with IgG 2 deficiency. Nihon Rinsho Meneki Gakkai Kaishi 21(2):70–79
49. Alejandria MM, Lansang MA, Dans LF, Mantaring JB (2002) Intravenous immunoglobulin for treating sepsis and septic shock. Cochrane Database Syst Rev (1):CD001090. Review.
50. Laupland KB, Kirkpatrick AW, Delaney A (2007) Polyclonal intravenous immunoglobulin for the treatment of severe sepsis and septic shock in critically ill adults: A systematic review and meta-analysis. Crit Care Med 35(12):2686–2692
51. Hagiwara S, Iwasaka H, Hasegawa A, Asai N, Noguchi T (2008) High-dose intravenous immunoglobulin G improves systemic inflammation in a rat model of CLP-induced sepsis. Intensive Care Med 34(10):1812–1819
52. Kreymann KG, de Heer G, Nierhaus A, Kluge S (2007) Use of polyclonal immunoglobulins as adjunctive therapy for sepsis or septic shock. Crit Care Med 35(12):2677–2685
53. Leong H, Stachnik J, Bonk ME, Matuszewski KA (2008) Unlabeled uses of intravenous immune globulin. Am M Health-Syst Pharm 65(19):1815–1824
54. Provan D, Chapel HM, Sewell WA, O'Shaughnessy D, UK Immunoglobulin Expert Working Group (2008) Prescribing intravenous immunoglobulin: summary of Department of Health guidelines. BMJ 2008 (337):a1831
55. Estrella L, Foley ME, Cunningham-Rundles C (2007) X-linked agammaglobulinemia in a 10-year-old child: a case study. J Am Acad Nurse Pract 19(4):205–211
56. Dellinger RP, Levy MM, Carlet JM, et al (2008) Surviving Sepsis Campaign: international guidelines for management of severe sepsis and septic shock: 2008. Crit Care Med 36(4):1394–1396
57. Fitzharris P, Hurst M (2008) Commentary: Controversies in the Department of Health's clinical guidelines for immunoglobulin use. BMJ 337:a1851
58. Turgeon AF, Hutton B, Fergusson DA, McIntyre L, Tinmouth AA, Cameron DW, Hébert PC (2007) Meta-analysis: intravenous immunoglobulin in critically ill adult patients with sepsis. Ann Int Med 146(3):193–203

Coagulation Disorders in Sepsis

10

Marcel Schouten and Tom van der Poll

1 Introduction

Sepsis is an acquired clinical syndrome, with symptoms resulting from a systemic host response to infection [1]. Sepsis is the most common cause of death among hospitalized patients in noncardiac intensive care units and has instigated much preclinical and clinical research [2]. Recently, tremendous progress has been made in understanding the complex triad of infection, inflammation, and coagulation during sepsis.

It is now well established that in sepsis systemic inflammation leads to activation of the coagulation system and inhibition of anticoagulant mechanisms and fibrinolysis (see Fig. 1). Activation of coagulation and subsequent fibrin deposition may be essential parts of the host defense against infectious agents in an attempt to contain the invading microorganisms and the subsequent inflammatory response [3]. However, an exaggerated response can lead to a situation in which coagulation itself contributes to disease, in its most severe form leading to microvascular thrombosis and consumption of coagulation factors, a syndrome known as disseminated intravascular coagulation (DIC) [4]. DIC is a common feature in sepsis, particularly in septic shock where the incidence is between 30 and 50%, and it plays an important role in the development of multiple organ failure (MOF) [5].

One of the important hallmarks of sepsis is microvascular dysfunction in which endothelial activation and dysfunction play a pivotal role [6]. In infection and subsequent sepsis, components of the bacterial cell wall as well as host-derived mediators activate pattern recognition receptors on the endothelial surface [7, 8]. The endothelium responds to this with structural and, importantly, functional changes, such as increased vascular permeability. This results in redistribution of body fluid and edema, which contribute to hypovolemia and hypotension that are important signs of the sepsis syndrome [6]. In normal situations the endothelium functions as an antithrombotic surface, preventing inappropriate activation of coagulation on the cell membrane [9]. However, when in sepsis

T. van der Poll (✉)
Center for Infection and Immunity Amsterdam (CINIMA), Center for Experimental and Molecular Medicine (CEMM), Academic Medical Center, University of Amsterdam, Meibergdreef 9, room G2-130, 1105 AZ Amsterdam, The Netherlands
e-mail: t.vanderpoll@amc.uva.nl

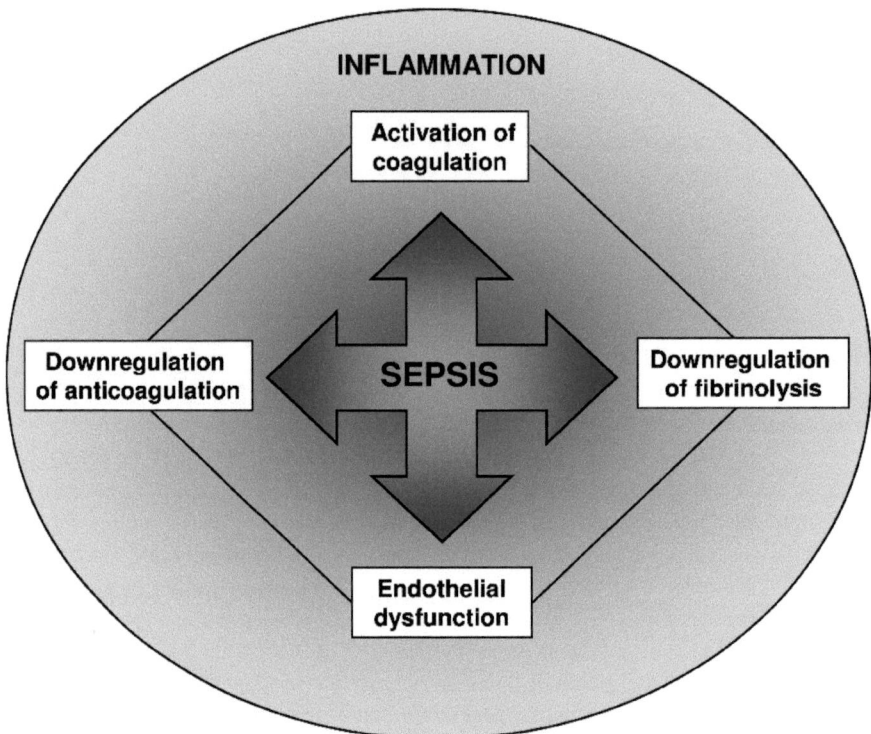

Fig. 1 Extensive crosstalk exists between coagulation, inflammation, and endothelial dysfunction in sepsis. Sepsis is characterized by endothelial dysfunction and inflammation-induced activation of coagulation with concurrent downregulation of anticoagulant systems and fibrinolysis. Inflammation-induced coagulation in turn modulates the inflammatory response in sepsis

the endothelium becomes activated, it transforms into a prothrombotic interface that is critically involved in the detrimental cascade leading to DIC and MOF (see Fig. 1).

It is becoming increasingly clear that inflammation not only leads to activation of the coagulation system, but that, vice versa, components of the coagulation system are also able to markedly modulate the inflammatory response [10]. Tissue factor (TF), thrombin, the protein C (PC) pathway, activators and inhibitors of fibrinolysis, and protease-activated receptors (PARs) have all been shown to play vital roles in the crosstalk between coagulation and inflammation in sepsis. In recent years, research in the field of coagulation and inflammation in sepsis has expanded its focus, now also covering, for example, microparticles (MPs) and platelets. In this chapter, the key players in inflammation-induced coagulation and coagulation-induced inflammation in sepsis are discussed with a special focus on the endothelium. Figure 2 provides an overview of the pathways discussed in this chapter.

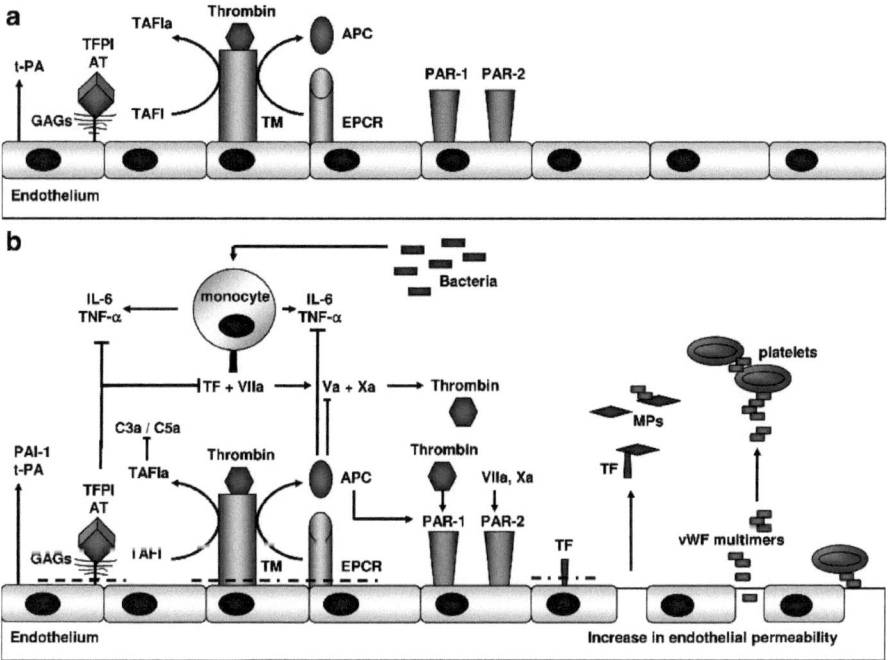

Fig. 2 The role of the endothelium in normal situations and in sepsis. **a** In normal situations the endothelial layer provides for an anticoagulant surface to prevent blood from clotting: The endothelium has the anticoagulant proteins tissue factor pathway inhibitor (*TFPI*) and antithrombin (*AT*) attached to its surface via glycosaminoglycans (*GAGs*) and secretes tissue-type plasminogen activator (*t-PA*), which promotes fibrinolysis. Moreover, the endothelium expresses thrombomodulin (*TM*) and the endothelial protein C receptor (*EPCR*), which support thrombin in generating the anticoagulant activated protein C (*APC*). TM-bound thrombin also activates thrombin activatable fibrinolysis inhibitor (*TAFI*). Protease-activated receptor (*PAR*)-1 and -2 are expressed on endothelial cells. **b** When in infection bacteria enter the bloodstream, systemic release of cytokines such as tumor necrosis factor (*TNF*)-α and interleukin (*IL*)-6 by, for example, monocytes leads to endothelial activation and dysfunction, increased endothelial permeability, and secretion of microparticles (*MPs*). Coagulation is activated by induction of tissue factor (*TF*) on monocytes and MPs and possibly also on endothelium which through assembly with factor (F)VII(a) results in activation of FV and FX and subsequent thrombin generation. The release of von Willebrand factor (*vWF*) multimers adds to platelet adhesion to the subendothelial surface and platelet aggregation. The anticoagulant proteins TFPI, AT, EPCR, and TM are cleaved from the endothelium and are impaired in action. Moreover, APC and AT are consumed. Fibrinolysis is impaired due to a rise in plasminogen activator inhibitor type-1 (*PAI-1*), which outweighs a rise in t-PA, and complement activation is enhanced by loss of activation of TAFI, which normally inhibits complement factor C3a and C5a and bradykinin activity. TF-FVIIa, FXa, and thrombin exert proinflammatory activity by cleaving PARs on the endothelium, and APC cleaves PAR-1 in an EPCR-dependent manner and hereby modulates inflammation

2
Activation of Coagulation

2.1
Tissue Factor

The pivotal initiator of inflammation-induced activation of coagulation is TF. TF initiates coagulation by catalyzing, in a newly formed complex with factor (F)VII(a), the conversion of the zymogens FIX and FX into active proteases, which in turn enhance the activation of FX and prothrombin, respectively. Prothrombin is converted to thrombin, which then converts fibrinogen to fibrin.

TF is present in all blood tissue barriers, so that coagulation can quickly be initiated when the endothelial barrier is disrupted, but it is normally not present in the vasculature [11]. In inflammatory conditions, however, TF is also induced, for example, by cytokines and C-reactive protein, in the circulatory system, predominantly on monocytes and macrophages [12]. This "inducible" TF is stimulated by the presence of platelets and granulocytes in a P-selectin-dependent manner [13]. The post-translational mechanism by which circulating TF activity is regulated is through so-called encryption and decryption, reflecting processes of self-association and -dissociation, respectively [14]. While the encrypted form of TF is inactive, the decrypted form exerts procoagulant activity. Recently, alternatively spliced TF (lacking exon 5) was discovered as a soluble form of TF, which freely circulates in blood and may exert procoagulant activity, expanding the concept of "circulating TF" by a further element [15]. Alternatively spliced TF is released from endothelial cells upon stimulation with proinflammatory cytokines [16].

In in vitro conditions, different cytokines such as tumor necrosis factor (TNF)-α and interleukin (IL)-1β induce TF on endothelial cells, but whether this also occurs to a relevant extent in vivo is still unclear [17]. Studies in baboons infused intravenously with *Escherichia (E.) coli* have suggested that TF is indeed expressed in the vascular wall during sepsis, especially in areas exposed to disturbed blood flow [18]. In contrast, TF was not detectable in endothelial cells from rabbits subjected to the generalized Shwartzman reaction by injection of two subsequent doses of lipopolysaccharide (LPS); moreover, immunohistochemical staining for TF failed to detect endothelial TF in rabbits administered with LPS [19].

The importance of inflammation-induced activation of coagulation by the TF-FVIIa complex is substantiated by experiments in nonhuman primates and human volunteers demonstrating that blocking of TF-FVIIa activity in *E coli* bacteremia or endotoxemia completely abrogated coagulation activation and – in lethal models – prevented DIC and mortality [20–23].

2.2
Microparticles

MPs are circulating cell fragments that are derived from activated or apoptotic cells. They contain significant amounts of surface-exposed negatively charged phospholipids that are essential for amplifying thrombin generation. As such, they are anticipated to contribute to a procoagulant state. Many different cell types have been shown to shed MPs, for example, monocytes, granulocytes, platelets, and endothelial cells [24].

MPs can also express TF on their surface: In human endotoxemia an increase in TF-containing MPs of up to 800% has been observed [25]. Moreover, TF and associated procoagulant activity have been detected on MPs derived from granulocytes and platelets in patients with meningococcal sepsis [26]. Monocyte-derived MPs have been shown to express TF after stimulation with LPS [27]. More recently, it was described that TF on monocyte-derived MPs is enhanced by platelets in a P-selectin-dependent manner [28]. P-selectin can also be expressed by endothelial cells when they are activated by thrombin. Indeed, MPs derived from TNF-α-stimulated human umbilical vein endothelial cells (HUVECs) induced coagulation in a TF-FVIIa-dependent way in vitro [29]. Moreover, endothelial MPs were shown to express von Willebrand factor (vWF) binding sites and to express ultralarge vWF-multimers, which potently promote the formation of platelet aggregates and increase their stability [30]. Endothelium-derived MPs have been detected in normal human blood and their levels were increased in patients with a coagulation abnormality characterized by the presence of lupus anticoagulant [31]. Whether endothelial MPs are also elevated in sepsis and indeed play a procoagulant role in this condition still needs to be determined.

2.3
Platelets and von Willebrand Factor

Platelets are involved in the pathophysiology of sepsis as marked by the frequent occurrence of thrombocytopenia in sepsis [32]. Platelets can be activated in sepsis, either directly by endotoxin or by proinflammatory cytokines [33, 34]. Platelets can also be activated by coagulation proteases such as thrombin, and when activated they secrete proinflammatory proteins and growth factors which contribute to inflammation. The negatively charged outer membrane surface of activated platelets provides an ideal surface for coagulation to take place on. Hence activated platelets can play an important role in inflammation-induced coagulation. As described above, platelets also interact with monocyte-derived MPs in a P-selectin-dependent manner and thereby enhance TF expression on MPs [28].

Platelets form platelet clots on a damaged endothelial layer. A first step in this process is adhesion by binding to vWF that is bound to collagen in the subendothelial layer. vWF also plays a role in subsequent platelet aggregation. vWF is produced predominantly by endothelial cells and when endothelium is activated or injured, vWF is released from preformed stores into the circulation. As such, vWF levels are generally accepted as a marker of endothelial injury [35]. In HUVECs various proinflammatory cytokines induce the release of ultralarge vWF multimers – which are very potent platelet aggregators – and moreover inhibit vWF cleavage by ADAMTS-13 [36]. Levels of vWF antigen are increased in sepsis and decreased levels of ADAMTS-13 have indeed been linked to a poor prognosis in sepsis [37]. The endothelium can thus contribute to platelet adhesion and aggregation in sepsis in various ways; by releasing vWF, especially ultralarge vWF multimers, and also indirectly by exposing subendothelial collagenous surfaces on which platelets can adhere in a vWF-dependent manner.

3
Impairment of Anticoagulant Systems

Under physiological conditions anticoagulant systems are continuously active to prevent blood from clotting on the endothelial cell surface [9]. The endothelium plays a key function in maintaining this anticoagulant condition. Blood clotting is controlled by three major anticoagulant endothelium-associated proteins: TF pathway inhibitor (TFPI), antithrombin, and activated PC (APC) [38].

3.1
Tissue Factor Pathway Inhibitor

TFPI is a serine protease inhibitor that is secreted mainly by endothelial cells [9]. TFPI inhibits the activation of FX to FXa by the TF-FVIIa complex. TFPI is normally attached to the endothelium via proteoglycans (PGs). which are glycosaminoglycans (GAGs) bound to a core protein, that facilitate its TF-FVIIa-FX-inhibiting properties on the endothelial surface [39]. In sepsis proinflammatory cytokines reduce the synthesis of GAGs on the endothelial surface, which likely impacts on TFPI function. Although reports on TFPI activity in situations of TF-induced coagulation have yielded contradictory results, an increase in plasma TFPI levels in meningococcal sepsis has been associated with more severe coagulation and mortality, supporting the hypothesis that TFPI works less efficiently when it is not attached to the endothelium [40].

The role of endogenous TFPI in anticoagulation in sepsis is illustrated by the fact that depletion of TFPI sensitized rabbits to LPS-induced DIC and the generalized Shwartzman reaction [41]. Conversely, administration of TFPI attenuated consumptive coagulopathy and improved survival in septic primates [42]. Administration of recombinant human TFPI prevented coagulation activation during human endotoxemia [20] and was able to attenuate coagulation activation in patients with severe sepsis, although this intervention did not result in a reduced mortality [43].

3.2
Antithrombin and Heparin

Antithrombin predominantly inhibits FXa and thrombin and also has inhibitory properties toward TF-FVIIa and FIXa. The anticoagulant properties of antithrombin have been shown extensively in vivo [44]. For example, treatment with antithrombin inhibited the procoagulant and hyperinflammatory response and, moreover, improved survival during severe sepsis in the baboon [45, 46]. Infusion of antithrombin dose-dependently reduced TF-triggered coagulation and ameliorated IL-6 production in a human model of endotoxemia [47]. Apart from its anticoagulant activities, antithrombin has been described to possess direct anti-inflammatory activity. For example, antithrombin decreased ischemia-reperfusion injury in the rat liver by increasing the hepatic level of prostacyclin and reducing leukocyte rolling on the endothelium [48, 49]. However, in sepsis, antithrombin levels are markedly decreased due to a combination of impaired synthesis, degradation, and – quantitatively the most important – consumption due to ongoing thrombin generation [38].

The anticoagulant activities of antithrombin are normally accelerated to a large extent by heparin-like GAGs, such as heparan sulfate (HS). Proinflammatory cytokines reduce the synthesis of GAGs on the endothelial surface. This contributes to reduced antithrombin function in sepsis. Of note, intravenous infusion of antithrombin did not alter mortality in patients with sepsis in a large multinational trial; however, in this population, a possible antithrombin effect may have been obscured by concurrent heparin treatment, considering that heparin – which is a highly sulfated version of HS – like soluble GAGs, is able to antagonize the anti-inflammatory and microcirculatory effects of antithrombin [50, 51].

While the synthesis of GAGs is reduced by proinflammatory cytokines, HSPGs specifically can be upregulated in inflammatory conditions [52]. HSPGs have been shown to facilitate leukocyte adhesion to the inflamed endothelium, to stimulate endothelial transcytosis and subsequent presentation of chemokines, which is important for the production of integrins that tighten leukocyte binding to the endothelium, and, moreover, to facilitate leukocyte transmigration through the vessel wall [53]. This implies that HSPGs could play an important proinflammatory role in sepsis. Therefore, administered heparin could in contrast play an anti-inflammatory role by interfering in the interaction between leukocytes and endothelial HSPGs [54].

3.3
The Protein C System

The PC system provides important control of coagulation by virtue of the capacity of APC to proteolytically inactivate the coagulation cofactors FVa and FVIIIa. APC is generated by thrombomodulin(TM)-bound thrombin. TM is present on the vascular endothelium in high concentrations, mainly in the microcirculation. The activation of PC to APC by TM-bound thrombin is augmented by the presence of the endothelial PC receptor (EPCR) [55]. TM-bound thrombin is efficiently inhibited by antithrombin and PC inhibitor. As a consequence, TM inhibits coagulation in various ways; by generating the anticoagulant APC, by accelerating the inhibition of thrombin, as well as by preventing thrombin from exerting its procoagulant properties on fibrinogen and platelets.

During sepsis the PC system is impaired as a result of decreased production of PC by the liver, increased consumption of PC, and decreased activation of PC by lower expression of TM on endothelial cells [10]. TM expression can be downregulated by inflammatory mediators such as TNF-α [56]. Additionally, LPS has been shown to stimulate neutrophil activation on the endothelial surface, leading to the release of elastase, which cleaves TM from the endothelium. This results in a rise in soluble TM, which is much less active than endothelium-bound TM, given the fact that it has no EPCR as cofactor on its side [57]. Moreover, neutrophils release oxidants that have been shown to oxidize TM, leaving behind a less active protein [58]. In patients with severe meningococcal sepsis, downregulation of TM and consequent impaired PC-activation were confirmed in vivo by immunohistochemistry [59]. Like TM, EPCR has also been shown to be cleaved from the endothelial surface, resulting in higher levels of soluble EPCR in sepsis [60]. It should be noted, however, that in a study that investigated soluble TM and soluble EPCR on the one hand and coagulation and survival in sepsis on the other hand, plasma levels of both soluble TM and soluble EPCR did not correlate with F1 + 2/APC ratios, which is a marker for the procoagulant state. Moreover, levels of both soluble TM and EPCR did not differ between survivors and nonsurvivors, indicating that the precise relationship between these soluble proteins and coagulation as well as outcome in sepsis has not been completely elucidated [57].

Several preclinical and clinical studies have supported the anticoagulant potency of the PC system in vivo. Infusion of APC into septic baboons prevented hypercoagulability and death, while inhibition of PC activation exacerbated the response to a lethal *E. coli* infusion and converted a sublethal model produced by an LD_{10} dose into a lethal DIC-associated model [61]. Treatment of baboons with an anti-EPCR monoclonal antibody was also associated with an exacerbation of a sublethal *E. coli* infection to lethal sepsis with DIC [62], and interference with the bioavailability of protein S (PS), an important cofactor for the anticoagulant functions of APC, resulted in similar changes [63]. Lastly, administration of recombinant human APC ameliorated coagulation and IL-6 levels in patients with severe sepsis and also reduced absolute mortality by 6% [64].

4
Impairment of Fibrinolysis

Homeostasis is further controlled by the fibrinolytic system, of which the end-product plasmin breaks down fibrin clots. Plasmin is generated from plasminogen by different proteases, most notably tissue-type plasminogen activator (t-PA) and urokinase-type (u-) PA. The main inhibitor of the PAs is PA inhibitor type 1 (PAI-1), which is produced by the endothelium and the liver and binds to t-PA and u-PA. In inflammatory states, the first fibrinolytic response is a release of t-PA and u-PA that is stored inside endothelial cells. This increase, however, is counteracted by a delayed but sustained increase in PAI-1 levels [65]. The net effect is impairment of fibrinolysis.

The importance of the fibrinolytic system for inflammation-induced coagulation in sepsis has been shown by experiments in genetically modified mice. Upon LPS administration, mice that were deficient for t-PA or u-PA had more fibrin deposition in their organs than wild-type mice, while the opposite held true for PAI-1-deficient mice [66]. As the main producer of both profibrinolytic factors and PAI-1, the endothelium plays an obvious role in fibrinolysis in sepsis.

5
Coagulation-Induced Inflammation

Inflammation not only leads to activation of coagulation, coagulation in turn also influences inflammation [10]. For example, heterozygously PC-deficient mice demonstrated higher levels of proinflammatory cytokines and increased neutrophil invasion in their lungs after intraperitoneal injection with endotoxin [67]. Conversely, APC attenuates inflammation by, for example, inhibiting monocyte expression of TNF-α, NFκB translocation, cytokine signaling, TNF-α-induced upregulation of cell surface leukocyte adhesion molecules, and leukocyte-endothelial cell interactions in vitro [68, 69]. TM also exerts anti-inflammatory effects at multiple levels. Firstly, TM is essential for the activation of PC to APC. Secondly, TM binds thrombin, thereby preventing it from exerting proinflammatory properties (see below). Thirdly, TM-bound thrombin also activates thrombin activatable fibrinolysis inhibitor (TAFI), which has been demonstrated to inhibit complement factor C3a and C5a and bradykinin activity [70]. Furthermore, the lectin domain of TM likely plays a direct role in the orchestration of inflammatory reactions: Genetically modified mice that lack the N-terminal lectin-like domain of TM displayed increased neutrophil recruitment to the lungs and diminished survival in a model of intravenously administered endotoxin [71]. The anti-inflammatory properties of antithrombin and heparin were already described earlier in this chapter in Sect. 3.2.

Multiple interactions also exist between mediators of the fibrinolytic system and inflammation. Fibrinolytic activators and inhibitors may modulate the inflammatory response by their effect on inflammatory cell recruitment and migration. For instance, u-PAR, the receptor for u-PA, mediates leukocyte adhesion to the vascular wall and extracellular matrix components and its expression on leukocytes is strongly associated with their migratory and tissue-invasive potential [72]. This is illustrated in a mouse model of bacterial pneumonia in which u-PAR-deficient mice displayed a profoundly reduced neutrophil influx into the pulmonary compartment [73]. Plasma concentrations of the fibrinolysis inhibitor PAI-1 are strongly elevated in patients with sepsis, and the level of PAI-1 is highly predictive of an unfavorable outcome [74]. It remains to be established whether the elevated PAI-1 levels are only indicative of a strong inflammatory response of the host, or indeed have any pathophysiological significance. Findings that a sequence variation in the gene encoding PAI-1 influences the development of septic shock in patients and relatives of patients with meningococcal infection have provided circumstantial evidence that PAI-1 might play a functional role in the host response to bacterial infection [75]. However, recent studies using PAI-1-deficient mice and mice with transiently enhanced expression of PAI-1 have pointed to a protective rather than a detrimental role of this mediator in severe Gram-negative pneumonia and sepsis [76].

5.1
Protease-Activated Receptors

In the crosstalk between coagulation and inflammation, protease-activated receptors (PARs) seem to play a pivotal role [77]. The PAR family consists of four members, PAR-1 to PAR-4, that are localized in the vasculature on different cell types such as endothelial cells, mononuclear cells, and platelets [78]. On endothelial cells, all four PARs have been identified [79]. PARs serve as their own ligand: proteolytic cleavage, for example, by a coagulation protease, leads to exposure of a neo-amino terminus, which serves as a ligand for the same receptor, hereby initiating transmembrane signaling. All PARs have been shown to play a role in inflammation. For example, LPS and proinflammatory cytokines induced PAR-2 and PAR-4 expression in cultured endothelial cells, and LPS- and TNF-α-induced IL-6 production by cultured endothelial cells was enhanced by the activation of PAR-1 and PAR-2.

The TF-FVIIa–FXa complex can signal through PAR-1 and PAR-2 at concentrations that are physiologically achievable; in contrast, TF-FVIIa or FXa alone require supraphysiological doses to exert comparable effects [80]. Low concentrations of thrombin have been shown to activate PAR-1, whereas high concentrations also activate PAR-3 and PAR-4. In humans, thrombin activates platelets by cleavage of PAR-1 and PAR-4; in mice, however, thrombin activates platelets by cleavage of a PAR-3–PAR-4 complex [81]. Thrombin can induce the expression of proinflammatory cytokines and chemokines by endothelium by cleaving PAR-1 in vitro [82].

Much effort has been made to elucidate the mechanisms by which APC exerts its various anti-inflammatory properties: APC inhibits inflammation indirectly through reducing thrombin generation and, thereby, thrombin-induced inflammation via PARs. However, in primary endothelial cells, APC itself also signals through PAR-1 in an EPCR-dependent manner, which induces the expression of a number of genes that are known to downregulate proinflammatory signaling pathways and inhibit apoptosis. APC also promotes endothelial barrier enhancement in vitro in an EPCR- and PAR-1-dependent manner, a property which could be of special interest given the central role of loss of endothelial barrier function in sepsis [83, 84]. However, whether the anti-inflammatory, anti-apoptotic, and barrier-stabilizing properties of APC play an important role during sepsis in vivo, and whether these are indeed mediated by PAR-1, is still a matter of debate [85, 86].

Most probably, the activation of multiple PARs mediates the crosstalk between coagulation and inflammation during sepsis. This is underscored by a recent study showing that while inhibition of thrombin with hirudin – to inhibit thrombin signaling through PAR-1 and PAR-4 – or a deficiency in either PAR-1 or PAR-2 did not affect IL-6 or mortality in a murine LPS model, combining hirudin treatment with PAR-2 deficiency did reduce IL-6 expression and additionally increased survival [87]. The crosstalk between coagulation and inflammation is also likely to be influenced by the timing of PAR activation. Recently, Kaneider et al. showed that activation of PAR-1 is harmful during the early phases of endotoxemia and sepsis, facilitating pulmonary leak and DIC, but beneficial at later stages in a PAR-2-dependent way [88]. This intriguing switch of PAR-1 from an exacerbating to a protective receptor is consistent with studies showing that PAR-1 deficiency conferred no net survival benefit in models of endotoxemia and sepsis [87, 89]. These results, however, are not completely in agreement with a recent paper by Niessen et al., who found that PAR-1-deficient mice were protected against mortality in an LD_{80} model of endotoxemia [90]. They found a reduced late-stage inflammation in PAR-1-deficient mice as indicated by a reduction in IL-6 and IL-1β levels 12 h after LPS injection. Reconstitution of inflammation in PAR-1-deficient mice could be achieved by adoptive transfer of wild-type bone marrow or purified dendritic cells. In a series of elegant experiments, these authors showed that while in the early phase of endotoxemia coagulation and inflammation do not interact, at later stages there appears to be a tight interaction between coagulation and inflammation, which is driven by the interaction between thrombin and PAR-1, more specifically PAR-1 that is expressed by dendritic cells [90].

6
Conclusions

There is ample evidence that activation of coagulation and downregulation of anticoagulation and fibrinolysis are prominent features of the proinflammatory condition in sepsis. The endothelium plays an important role in these sequelae. The procoagulant state in sepsis in turn enhances inflammation, presumably especially through activation of PARs. In the near future, a further delineation of the role of the multiple PARs and their interaction with coagulation proteases will probably contribute significantly to our understanding of the crosstalk between coagulation and inflammation in sepsis.

Abbreviations

APC	Activated protein C
AT	Antithrombin
DIC	Disseminated intravascular coagulation
E. coli	*Escherichia coli*
EPCR	Endothelial protein C receptor
HUVEC	Human umbilical vein endothelial cell
FV(a)	Coagulation factor V (activated)
FVII(a)	Coagulation factor VII (activated)
FX(a)	Coagulation factor X (activated)
FXI(a)	Coagulation factor XI (activated)
GAG	Glycosaminoglycan
HS	Heparan sulfate
IL	Interleukin
LPS	Lipopolysaccharide
MOF	Multiple organ failure
MP	Microparticle
PAI-1	Plasminogen activator inhibitor type 1
PAR	Protease-activated receptor
PC	Protein C
PG	Proteoglycan
PS	Protein S
TAFI	Thrombin activatable fibrinolysis inhibitor
TF	Tissue factor
TFPI	Tissue factor pathway inhibitor
TM	Thrombomodulin
TNF-α	Tumor necrosis factor-α
t-PA	Tissue-type plasminogen activator
u-PA	Urokinase-type plasminogen activator
u-PAR	Urokinase-type plasminogen activator receptor
vWF	von Willebrand factor

References

1. Cohen J (2002) The immunopathogenesis of sepsis. Nature 420:885–891
2. Angus DC, Linde-Zwirble WT, Lidicker J, Clermont G, Carcillo J, and Pinsky MR (2001) Epidemiology of severe sepsis in the United States: Analysis of incidence, outcome, and associated costs of care. Crit Care Med 29:1303–1310
3. Opal SM and Esmon CT (2003) Bench-to-bedside review: functional relationships between coagulation and the innate immune response and their respective roles in the pathogenesis of sepsis. Crit Care 7:23–38
4. Levi M and Ten Cate H (1999) Disseminated intravascular coagulation. N Engl J Med 341: 586–592
5. Dhainaut JF, Yan SB, Joyce DE, Pettila V, Basson B, Brandt JT, Sundin DP, and Levi M (2004) Treatment effects of drotrecogin alfa (activated) in patients with severe sepsis with or without overt disseminated intravascular coagulation. J Thromb Haemost 2:1924–1933
6. Aird WC (2003) The role of the endothelium in severe sepsis and multiple organ dysfunction syndrome. Blood 101:3765–3777
7. Henneke P and Golenbock D T (2002) Innate immune recognition of lipopolysaccharide by endothelial cells. Crit Care Med 30:S207–S213
8. Zhang FX, Kirschning CJ, Mancinelli R, Xu XP, Jin YP, Faure E, Mantovani A, Rothe M, Muzio M, and Arditi M (1999) Bacterial lipopolysaccharide activates nuclear factor-kappa B through interleukin-1 signaling mediators in cultured human dermal endothelial cells and mononuclear phagocytes. J Biol Chem 274:7611–7614
9. Bombeli T, Müller M, and Häberli A (1997) Anticoagulant properties of the vascular endothelium. Thromb Haemost 77:408–423
10. Levi M, Van der Poll T, and Büller H R (2004) Bidirectional relation between inflammation and coagulation. Circulation 109:2698–2704
11. Camerer E, Kolsto A B, and Prydz H (1996) Cell biology of tissue factor, the principal initiator of blood coagulation. Thromb Res 81:1–41
12. Osterud B and Flaegstad T (1983) Increased tissue thromboplastin activity in monocytes of patients with meningococcal infection: related to an unfavourable prognosis. Thromb Haemost 49:5–7
13. Osterud B (1998) Tissue factor expression by monocytes: regulation and pathophysiological roles. Blood Coagulat Fibrinol 9:S9–S14
14. Monroe DM and Key NS (2007) The tissue factor-factor VIIa complex: procoagulant activity, regulation, and multitasking. J Thromb Haemost 5:1097–1105
15. Bogdanov V, Pyo R T, Taubman M B, and Nemerson Y (2002) Identification of alternatively spliced murine tissue factor mRNA and protein. Circulation 106:39–39
16. Szotowski B, Antoniak S, Poller W, Schultheiss H P, and Rauch U (2005) Procoagulant soluble tissue factor is released from endothelial cells in response to inflammatory cytokines. Circulation Res 96:1233–1239
17. Bevilacqua MP, Pober JS, Majeau GR, Fiers W, Cotran RS, and Gimbrone MA, Jr. (1986) Recombinant tumor necrosis factor induces procoagulant activity in cultured human vascular endothelium: characterization and comparison with the actions of interleukin 1. Proc Natl Acad Sci U S A 83:4533–4537
18. Lupu C, Westmuckett AD, Peer G, Ivanciu L, Zhu H, Taylor FB, and Lupu F (2005) Tissue factor-dependent coagulation is preferentially up-regulated within arterial branching areas in a baboon model of *Escherichia coli* sepsis. Am J Pathol 167:1161–1172
19. Erlich J, Fearns C, Mathison J, Ulevitch R J, and Mackman N (1999) Lipopolysaccharide induction of tissue factor expression in rabbits. Infect Immun 67:2540–2546
20. De Jonge E, Dekkers PEP, Creasey AA, Hack CE, Paulson SK, Karim A, Kesecioglu J, Levi M, Van Deventer SJH, and Van der Poll T (2000) Tissue factor pathway inhibitor dose-dependently

inhibits coagulation activation without influencing the fibrinolytic and cytokine response during human endotoxemia. Blood 95:1124–1129
21. De Pont ACJM, Moons AHM, de Jonge E, Meijers JCM, Vlasuk GP, Rote WE, Büller HR, Van der Poll T, and Levi M (2004) Recombinant nematode anticoagulant protein c2, an inhibitor of tissue factor/factor VIIa, attenuates coagulation and the interleukin-10 response in human endotoxemia. J Thromb Haemost 2:65–70
22. Levi M, Ten Cate H, Bauer KA, Van der Poll T, Edgington TS, Büller HR, Van Deventer SJH, Hack CE, Ten Cate JW, and Rosenberg RD (1994) Inhibition of endotoxin-induced activation of coagulation and fibrinolysis by pentoxifylline or by a monoclonal antitissue factor antibody in chimpanzees. J Clin Investig 93:114–120
23. Taylor FB, Chang A, Ruf W, Morrissey JH, Hinshaw L, Catlett R, Blick K, and Edgington TS (1991) Lethal *Escherichia coli* septic shock is prevented by blocking tissue factor with monoclonal-antibody. Circulatory Shock 33:127–134
24. Berckmans RJ, Nieuwland R, Boing AN, Romijn FPHT, Hack CE, and Sturk A (2001) Cell-derived microparticles circulate in healthy humans and support low grade thrombin generation. Thromb Haemost 85:639–646
25. Aras O, Shet A, Bach RR, Hysjulien JL, Slungaard A, Hebbel RP, Escolar G, Jilma B, and Key NS (2004) Induction of microparticle- and cell-associated intravascular tissue factor in human endotoxemia. Blood 103:4545–4553
26. Nieuwland R, Berckmans RJ, McGregor S, Boing AN, Romijn FPHT, Westendorp RGJ, Hack CE, and Sturk A (2000) Cellular origin and procoagulant properties of microparticles in meningococcal sepsis. Blood 95:930–935
27. Satta N, Toti F, Feugeas O, Bohbot A, Dacharyprigent J, Eschwege V, Hedman H, and Freyssinet JM (1994) Monocyte vesiculation is a possible mechanism for dissemination of membrane-associated procoagulant activities and adhesion molecules After stimulation by lipopolysaccharide. J Immunol 153:3245–3255
28. Del Conde I, Shrimpton CN, Thiagarajan P, and Lopez JA (2005) Tissue-factor-bearing microvesicles arise from lipid rafts and fuse with activated platelets to initiate coagulation. Blood 106:1604–1611
29. Combes V, Simon AC, Grau GE, Arnoux D, Camoin L, Sabatier F, Mutin M, Sanmarco M, Sampol J, and Dignat-George F (1999) In vitro generation of endothelial microparticles and possible prothrombotic activity in patients with lupus anticoagulant. J Clin Invest 104: 93–102
30. Jy W, Jimenez JJ, Cheng PY, Mauro LM, Horstman LL, Ahn ER, Bidot CJ, and Ahn YS (2004) Endothelial microparticles (EMP) bind and complex with unusually-large multimers of von Willebrand factor (ULvWf) and act as potent inducers of platelet adhesion and aggregation. Blood 104:997A–998A
31. Dignat-George F, Camoin-Jau L, Sabatier F, Arnoux D, Anfosso F, Bardin N, Veit V, Combes V, Gentile S, Moal V, Sanmarco M, and Sampol J (2004) Endothelial microparticles: a potential contribution to the thrombotic complications of the antiphospholipid syndrome. Thromb Haemost 91:667–673
32. Akca S, Haji-Michael P, De Mendonca A, Suter P, Levi M, and Vincent JL (2002) Time course of platelet counts in critically ill patients. Crit Care Med 30:753–756
33. Zielinski T, Wachowicz B, Saluk-Juszczak J, and Kaca W (2002) Polysaccharide part of *Proteus mirabilis* lipopolysaccharide may be responsible for the stimulation of platelet adhesion to collagen. Platelets 13:419–424
34. Zimmerman GA, McIntyre TM, Prescott SM, and Stafforini DM (2002) The platelet-activating factor signaling system and its regulators in syndromes of inflammation and thrombosis. Crit Care Med 30:S294–S301
35. Reinhart K, Bayer O, Brunkhorst F, and Meisner M (2002) Markers of endothelial damage in organ dysfunction and sepsis. Crit Care Med 30:S302–S312

36. Bernardo A, Ball C, Nolasco L, Moake J F, and Dong J F (2004) Effects of inflammatory cytokines on the release and cleavage of the endothelial cell-derived ultralarge von Willebrand factor multimers under flow. Blood 104:100–106
37. Martin K, Borgel D, Lerolle N, Feys H B, Trinquart L, Vanhoorelbeke K, Deckmyn H, Legendre P, Diehl J L, and Baruch D (2007) Decreased ADAMTS-13 (A disintegrin-like and metalloprotease with thrombospondin type 1 repeats) is associated with a poor prognosis in sepsis-induced organ failure. Crit Care Med 35:2375–2382
38. Levi M and Van der Poll T (2005) Two-way interactions between inflammation and coagulation. Trends Cardiovasc Med 15:254–259
39. Ott I, Miyagi Y, Miyazaki K, Heeb MJ, Müller BM, Rao LVM, and Ruf W (2000) Reversible regulation of tissue factor-induced coagulation by glycosylphosphatidylinositol-anchored tissue factor pathway inhibitor. Arterioscler Thromb Vasc Biol 20:874–882
40. Brandtzaeg P, Sandset PM, Joo GB, Ovstebo R, Abildgaard U, and Kierulf P (1989) The quantitative association of plasma endotoxin, antithrombin, protein C, extrinsic pathway inhibitor and fibrinopeptide A in systemic meningococcal disease. Thromb Res 55:459–470
41. Sandset PM, Warncramer BJ, Maki SL, and Rapaport SI (1991) Immunodepletion of extrinsic pathway inhibitor sensitizes rabbits to endotoxin-induced intravascular coagulation and the generalized Shwartzman reaction. Blood 78:1496–1502
42. Creasey AA, Chang ACK, Feigen L, Wun TC, Taylor FB, and Hinshaw LB (1993) Tissue factor pathway inhibitor reduces mortality from *Escherichia Coli* septic shock. J Clin Invest 91:2850–2860
43. Abraham E, Reinhart K, Opal S, Demeyer I, Doig C, Rodriguez AL, Beale R, Svoboda P, Laterre PF, Simon S, Light B, Spapen H, Stone J, Seibert A, Peckelsen C, De Deyne C, Postier R, Pettila V, Artigas A, Percell SR, Shu V, Zwingelstein C, Tobias J, Poole L, Stolzenbach JC, and Creasey AA (2003) Efficacy and safety of tifacogin (recombinant tissue factor pathway inhibitor) in severe sepsis: a randomized controlled trial. JAMA 290:238–247
44. Dickneite G (1998) Preclinical evaluation of antithrombin III in experimental sepsis and DIC. Blood 92:357A
45. Minnema MC, Chang AC, Jansen PM, Lubbers YT, Pratt BM, Whittaker BG, Taylor FB, Hack CE, and Friedman B (2000) Recombinant human antithrombin III improves survival and attenuates inflammatory responses in baboons lethally challenged with *Escherichia coli*. Blood 95:1117–1123
46. Taylor FB Jr, Emerson TE Jr, Jordan R, Chang AK, and Blick KE (1988) Antithrombin-III prevents the lethal effects of *Escherichia coli* infusion in baboons. Circ Shock 26:227–235
47. Leitner JM, Firbas C, Mayr FB, Reiter RA, Steinlechner B, and Jilma B (2006) Recombinant human antithrombin inhibits thrombin formation and interleukin 6 release in human endotoxemia. Clin Pharmacol Therapeut 79:23–34
48. Harada N, Okajima K, Kushimoto S, Isobe H, and Tanaka K (1999) Antithrombin reduces ischemia/reperfusion injury of rat liver by increasing the hepatic level of prostacyclin. Blood 93:157–164
49. Ostrovsky L, Woodman RC, Payne D, Teoh D, and Kubes P (1997) Antithrombin III prevents and rapidly reverses leukocyte recruitment in ischemia/reperfusion. Circulation 96:2302–2310
50. Horie S, Ishii H, and Kazama M (1990) Heparin-like glycosaminoglycan is a receptor for antithrombin III-dependent but not for thrombin-dependent prostacyclin production in human endothelial cells. Thromb Res 59:895–904
51. Warren BL, Eid A, Singer P, Pillay SS, Carl P, Novak I, Chalupa P, Atherstone A, Penzes I, Kubler A, Knaub S, Keinecke HO, Heinrichs H, Schindel F, Juers M, Bone RC, and Opal SM (2001) High-dose antithrombin III in severe sepsis – a randomized controlled trial. J Am Med Assoc 286:1869–1878
52. Gotte M (2003) Syndecans in inflammation. FASEB J 17:575–591
53. Parish CR (2006) The role of heparan sulphate in inflammation. Nat Rev Immunol 6:633–643

54. Xie X, Rivier AS, Zakrzewicz A, Bernimoulin M, Zeng XL, Wessel HP, Schapira M, and Spertini O (2000) Inhibition of selectin-mediated cell adhesion and prevention of acute inflammation by nonanticoagulant sulfated saccharides – studies with carboxyl-reduced and sulfated heparin and with trestatin A sulfate. J Biol Chem 275:34818–34825
55. Esmon CT (2003) The protein C pathway. Chest 124:26S–32S
56. Conway EM and Rosenberg RD (1988) Tumor necrosis factor suppresses transcription of the thrombomodulin gene in endothelial cells. Mol Cell Biol 8:5588–5592
57. Liaw PC, Esmon CT, Kahnamoui K, Schmidt S, Kahnamoui S, Ferrell G, Beaudin S, Julian JA, Weitz JI, Crowther M, Loeb M, and Cook D (2004) Patients with severe sepsis vary markedly in their ability to generate activated protein C. Blood 104:3958–3964
58. Takano S, Kimura S, Ohdama S, and Aoki N (1990) Plasma thrombomodulin in health and diseases. Blood 76:2024–2029
59. Faust SN, Levin M, Harrison OB, Goldin RD, Lockhart MS, Kondaveeti S, Laszik Z, Esmon CT, and Heyderman RS (2001) Dysfunction of endothelial protein C activation in severe meningococcal sepsis. N Engl J Med 345:408–416
60. Xu J, Qu D, Esmon NL, and Esmon CT (2000) Metalloproteolytic release of endothelial cell protein C receptor. J Biol Chem 275:6038–6044
61. Taylor FB Jr, Chang A, Esmon CT, D'Angelo A, Vigano-D'Angelo S, and Blick KE (1987) Protein C prevents the coagulopathic and lethal effects of *Escherichia coli* infusion in the baboon. J Clin Invest 79:918–925
62. Taylor FB Jr, Stearns-Kurosawa DJ, Kurosawa S, Ferrell G, Chang AC, Laszik Z, Kosanke S, Peer G, and Esmon CT (2000) The endothelial cell protein C receptor aids in host defense against *Escherichia coli* sepsis. Blood 95:1680–1686
63. Taylor FB Jr, Chang AC, Peer GT, Mather T, Blick K, Catlett R, Lockhart MS, and Esmon CT (1991) DEGR-factor Xa blocks disseminated intravascular coagulation initiated by *Escherichia coli* without preventing shock or organ damage. Blood 78:364–368
64. Bernard GR, Vincent JL, Laterre PF, LaRosa SP, Dhainaut JF, Lopez-Rodriguez A, Steingrub JS, Garber GE, Helterbrand JD, Ely EW, and Fisher CJ Jr. (2001) Efficacy and safety of recombinant human activated protein C for severe sepsis. N Engl J Med 344:699–709
65. Van der Poll T, Levi M, Büller HR, Van Deventer SJ, De Boer JP, Hack CE, and Ten Cate JW (1991) Fibrinolytic response to tumor necrosis factor in healthy subjects. J Exp Med 174:729–732
66. Carmeliet P, Schoonjans L, Kieckens L, Ream B, Degen J, Bronson R, Devos R, Vandenoord JJ, Collen D, and Mulligan RC (1994) Physiological consequences of loss of plasminogen-activator gene-function in mice. Nature 368:419–424
67. Levi M, Dörffler-Melly J, Reitsma P, Büller H, Florquin S, Van der Poll T, and Carmeliet P (2003) Aggravation of endotoxin-induced disseminated intravascular coagulation and cytokine activation in heterozygous protein-C-deficient mice. Blood 101:4823–4827
68. Esmon CT (2005) The interactions between inflammation and coagulation. Br J Haematol 131:417–430
69. Van de Wouwer M, Collen D, and Conway EM (2004) Thrombomodulin-protein C-EPCR system: integrated to regulate coagulation and inflammation. Arterioscler Thromb Vasc Biol 24:1374–1383
70. Myles T, Nishimura T, Yun T H, Nagashima M, Morser J, Patterson AJ, Pearl RG, and Leung LL (2003) Thrombin activatable fibrinolysis inhibitor, a potential regulator of vascular inflammation. J Biol Chem 278:51059–51067
71. Conway EM, Van de Wouwer M, Pollefeyt S, Jurk K, Van Aken H, De Vriese A, Weitz JI, Weiler H, Hellings PW, Schaeffer P, Herbert JM, Collen D, and Theilmeier G (2002) The lectin-like domain of thrombomodulin confers protection from neutrophil-mediated tissue damage by suppressing adhesion molecule expression via nuclear factor kappaB and mitogen-activated protein kinase pathways. J Exp Med 196:565–577
72. Blasi F (1999) Proteolysis, cell adhesion, chemotaxis, and invasiveness are regulated by the u-PA-u-PAR-PAI-1 system. Thromb Haemost 82:298–304

73. Rijneveld AW, Levi M, Florquin S, Speelman P, Carmeliet P, and Van der Poll T (2002) Urokinase receptor is necessary for adequate host defense against pneumococcal pneumonia. J Immunol 168:3507–3511
74. Raaphorst J, Groeneveld ABJ, Bossink AW, and Hack CE (2001) Early inhibition of activated fibrinolysis predicts microbial infection, shock and mortality in febrile medical patients. Thromb Haemost 86:543–549
75. Hermans PW and Hazelzet JA (2005) Plasminogen activator inhibitor type 1 gene polymorphism and sepsis. Clin Infect Dis 41(Suppl 7):S453–S458
76. Renckens R, Roelofs JJTH, Bonta PI, Florquin S, de Vries CJM, Levi M, Carmeliet P, Van 't Veer C, and Van der Poll T (2007) Plasminogen activator inhibitor type 1 is protective during severe Gram-negative pneumonia. Blood 109:1593–1601
77. Ossovskaya VS and Bunnett NW (2004) Protease-activated receptors: Contribution to physiology and disease. Physiol Rev 84:579–621
78. Coughlin SR (2000) Thrombin signalling and protease-activated receptors. Nature 407:258–264
79. Bunnett NW (2006) Protease-activated receptors: how proteases signal to cells to cause inflammation and pain. Semin Thromb Hemost 32(Suppl 1):39–48
80. Ruf W, Dorfleutner A, and Riewald M (2003) Specificity of coagulation factor signaling. J Thromb Haemost 1:1495–1503
81. Nakanishi-Matsui M, Zheng YW, Sulciner DJ, Weiss EJ, Ludeman MJ, and Coughlin SR (2000) PAR3 is a cofactor for PAR4 activation by thrombin. Nature 404:609–613
82. Riewald M, Petrovan RJ, Donner A, Müller BM, and Ruf W (2002) Activation of endothelial cell protease activated receptor 1 by the protein C pathway. Science 296:1880–1882
83. Feistritzer C and Riewald M (2005) Endothelial barrier protection by activated protein C through PAR1-dependent sphingosine 1-phosphate receptor-1 crossactivation. Blood 105:3178–3184
84. Ludeman MJ, Kataoka H, Srinivasan Y, Esmon NL, Esmon CT, and Coughlin SR (2005) PAR1 cleavage and signaling in response to activated protein C and thrombin. J Biol Chem 280:13122–13128
85. Esmon CT (2005) Is APC activation of endothelial cell PAR1 important in severe sepsis?: No. J Thromb Haemost 3:1910–1911
86. Ruf W (2005) Is APC activation of endothelial cell PAR1 important in severe sepsis?: Yes. J Thromb Haemost 3:1912–1914
87. Pawlinski R, Pedersen B, Schabbauer G, Tencati M, Holscher T, Boisvert W, Andrade-Gordon P, Frank RD, and Mackman N (2004) Role of tissue factor and protease-activated receptors in a mouse model of endotoxemia. Blood 103:1342–1347
88. Kaneider NC, Leger AJ, Agarwal A, Nguyen N, Perides G, Derian C, Covic L, and Kuliopulos A (2007) "Role reversal" for the receptor PAR1 in sepsis-induced vascular damage. Nat Immunol 8(12):1303–1312
89. Camerer E, Cornelissen I, Kataoka H, Duong DN, Zheng YW, and Coughlin SR (2006) Roles of protease-activated receptors in a mouse model of endotoxemia. Blood 107:3912–3921
90. Niessen F, Schaffner F, Furlan-Freguia C, Pawlinski R, Bhattacharjee G, Chun J, Derian CK, Andrade-Gordon P, Rosen H, and Ruf W (2008) Dendritic cell PAR1-S1P3 signalling couples coagulation and inflammation. Nature 452:654–658

Antibiotics in Severe Sepsis: Which Combinations Work?

11

Tobias Welte

Every second patient who stays longer than 24 h in an intensive care unit (ICU) develops at the onset or at some point thereafter an infection [1]. Every fourth patient with such an infection will develop sepsis within the following 28 days. Sepsis remains the most frequent complication causing death in modern intensive care medicine [2]. The presence of sepsis not only increases mortality, but also results in a considerable rise in the overall costs of treatment [3].

The introduction of modern therapeutic practices (Overview 4) has reduced sepsis-related mortality from approximately 70% to around 50% during the last few years, although this figure is still considered unacceptably high. A recent study conducted by the German Network for Excellence in Sepsis (SepNet) evaluated the prevalence of sepsis within Germany, and found that it is in accordance with previously published American results [4].

1
Epidemiology and Microbiology

The occurrence of infection during admission to an ICU is associated with a definite rise in mortality within these units [5]. With the increasing severity of infection, the frequency of organ failure and the likelihood of ensuing treatment-refractory shock are markedly elevated, leading to a dramatic rise in mortality from severe sepsis and septic shock [6].

As a consequence of the aging of the population and medical advances (increasing surgical procedures in high-risk patients, the frequent use of immunosuppressive treatment in malignant and systemic disease), there is an inevitable increase in sepsis complications that must be contended with [3, 6]. In Germany, the prevalence of sepsis along with severe sepsis/septic shock has been estimated at 12.4 and 11%, respectively, which corresponds to an incidence of 76–110 cases per 100,000 of the population [6].

The most important sites of infection for either severe sepsis or septic shock are the lungs and the intra-abdominal cavity, with a lower incidence found in the urogenital

---

T. Welte (✉)
Department of Respiratory Medicine, Medizinische Hochschule Hannover
(Hannover Medical School), Carl-Neuberg-Strasse 1, D-30625 Hannover, Germany
e-mail: welte.tobias@mh-hannover.de

system, the skin, and soft tissue [6]. The primary focus of sepsis is not identified in approximately 5–10% of all sepsis cases, which are believed to be of staphylococcal origin.

The spectrum of anticipated pathogens is highly dependent on the source of infection. Community-acquired pneumonia (CAP) tends to be dominated by *Streptococcus pneumoniae* and *Legionella pneumophila*, whereas hospital-acquired pneumonia (HAP) and in particular ventilator-associated pneumonia (VAP) are more likely to be associated with staphylococci, enterobacteria (*Escherichia coli*, *Klebsiella*) and non-fermenters such as *Pseudomonas aeruginosa*, as well as other multiresistant pathogens such as *Acinetobacter* or *Stenotrophomonas maltophilia*.

In early-phase intra-abdominal infections, enterobacteria and anaerobes tend to dominate. However, in the course of the disease, particularly preceding tertiary peritonitis, multiresistant infections due to enterococci as well as candida predominate.

Skin and soft-tissue infections tend to be dominated by staphylococci (with a high rate of MRSA), anaerobic, and difficult-to-treat Gram-negative infections.

E. coli remains the predominant cause of urosepsis. In patients having previously received multiple antibiotics, *P. aeruginosa* plays an increasingly important role.

The origin of each sepsis, the expected clinical course, and the potential risk factors require consideration when determining the choice of suitable antibiotic strategies, particularly with regard to the necessity and nature of the combination therapy.

The prevalence of fungal infections, particularly in non-immunosuppressed patients, appears to be increasing [7]. There seem to be two fundamental reasons for this. First, the patients treated within the ICU environment are becoming increasingly older, partly due to the general aging of the population, but also through the ever more aggressive and sophisticated treatment employed for aging patient populations. While enormous medical advances have led to improved survival, this is associated with prolonged treatment within an intensive care setting. These cases involve the most seriously ill patients who tend to exhibit incumbent immunosuppression, paving the way perfectly for further fungal opportunistic infections. Another reason for such infections comes from the fact that there is virtually no longer ICU treatment without long periods of antibiotic exposure. The applied therapies often promote not only Candida, but also other multiresistant bacterial infections.

Both of these aspects, namely, the importance of the source of infection in terms of mortality, and the pathogen epidemiology, require careful consideration when planning appropriate antimicrobial therapy. There exists great variability within the epidemiology of infection. This is not just limited between different regions or countries, but considerable differences in resistance patterns of important pathogens are observed between different hospitals in the same town, and even between ICUs in the same hospital [8]. Every ICU should have statistics on the prevalence of pathogens and their resistance patterns, and these statistics should be reviewed every 6–12 months, depending on ward size.

2
Resistance Development

Since the mid-1990s a rapid increase in resistance of all the important pathogens against standard antibiotics has been observed. Noteworthy examples include methicillin-resistant *Staphylococcus aureus* (MRSA), vancomycin-resistant Enterococcus (VRE), the extended-spectrum beta-lactamases (ESBL) producing *E. coli* and *Klebsiella pneumoniae*, as well as ceftazidime, ciprofloxacin, or carbapenem-resistant *P. aeruginosa* [9]. Between times there have also been single case reports involving pathogens that failed to demonstrate sensitivity to any known class of antibiotics.

In the United States, a rise in multiresistant organisms has been observed even within outpatient populations over recent years, resulting from a rapid increase in the prevalence of so-called community-acquired MRSA (c-MRSA or ca-MRSA), mainly in the form of skin and soft-tissue infections. This unfortunately also reflects an increase in severe necrotizing pneumonia. On this issue, there is currently a large difference in prevalence between Europe and the United States, suggesting that existing American Guidelines can only be applied in Europe with respect to combination therapy.

The increasing incidence of antibiotic-associated pseudomembranous colitis (caused by *Clostridium difficile* toxin) in both outpatient (particularly in elderly and residential-care patients) and inpatient groups represents another relevant problem. In 70–80% of cases the colitis is related directly to the introduction of antibiotic treatment, while in the remaining patients, mainly in nursing homes and in the hospital, transmission between patients becomes a major problem. The causative antibiotics often included the usual underlying pathogen (clindamycin, cephalosporins, as well as the fluoroquinolones). In addition to the increasing incidence, certain *C. difficile* clones (O27, and recently O78) are beginning to demonstrate increased pathogenicity with detectable rises in both morbidity and mortality [10]. The detection of *C. difficile* toxin in combination with typical clinical features – profuse, nonbloody diarrhea – is today considered proof of the condition. The standard therapy consists of discontinuing the suspected causative antibiotic and commencing oral metronidazole at a dose of 400 mg four times daily. However, treatment failure tends to occur relatively frequently (10–20%), and in such cases oral vancomycin (125–250 mg, every 6 h) represents an acceptable alternative [11]. If oral administration is impossible, parenteral treatment with antibiotics exhibiting good intestinal penetration should be considered despite the accepted reduction in efficacy. Newer intravenous antibiotics such as tigecycline and linezolid, alongside metronidazole, should be considered in such cases. Vancomycin exhibits poor penetration in its parenteral form and is therefore considered unsuitable.

3
Treatment

The fundamental requirement of sepsis treatment is the successful cleansing of the focus of infection. Along with surgical debridement, the choice of adequate antimicrobial therapy for the duration of the illness must be decided. Unfortunately, only a few controlled studies exist that focus on anti-infective agents with different therapeutic regimes (escalation vs. de-escalation, mono vs. combination therapy) and treatment duration. Both, the pharmacodynamic and pharmacokinetic aspects have never been practically investigated until today. The treatment recommendations are therefore somewhat unclear in the various guidelines – either confined to generalized advice, or so broad that the myriad of named antimicrobial agents mean that no definitive advice can be derived for daily practice [36].

The predominant risk factor for increased mortality due to sepsis remains inadequate initial antibiotic therapy. This could be shown in a Spanish study, in which an increased mortality of almost 40% due to inappropriate initial treatment was demonstrated [12].

The term "adequate treatment" refers not only to the selection of the appropriate antibiotics, but also to the initiation of this treatment as early as possible.

A recently published retrospective observational study from Kumar and colleagues [13] examined the effect of delayed initiation of treatment in 2,154 patients with septic shock. They identified a 7% increase in mortality for every hour that initiation of treatment was delayed (Fig. 1). Even within the first "golden hour" a detectable difference was demonstrated. Patients receiving treatment within the first 30 min demonstrated an 82.7% survival rate, in comparison to 77.2% in those beginning treatment in the second half of this "golden hour."

The Kumar findings have been subsequently confirmed in another study. Blot et al. [14] studied patients with severe CAP, focusing on the effect of early measurement of oxygen saturation on survival. A direct correlation between the time of initial measurement of saturations and patient survival was identified, which was attributed entirely to the subsequent early initiation of antibiotic therapy.

This necessity for a rapid initiation of treatment generally compels the initial usage of broad-spectrum antibiotics, given that the earliest reliable microbiological results will only be available after 24–48 h. This problem is aggravated by the fact that in only 55% of outpatient-acquired infections, and only in 71% of nosocomial infections, was the causative organism successfully identified [15].

In patients with severe infections, diagnostic procedures should not lead to any delay in the initiation of treatment. In such cases further microbiological diagnosis – with the exception of taking two pairs of blood cultures – is therefore, as a general rule, not possible.

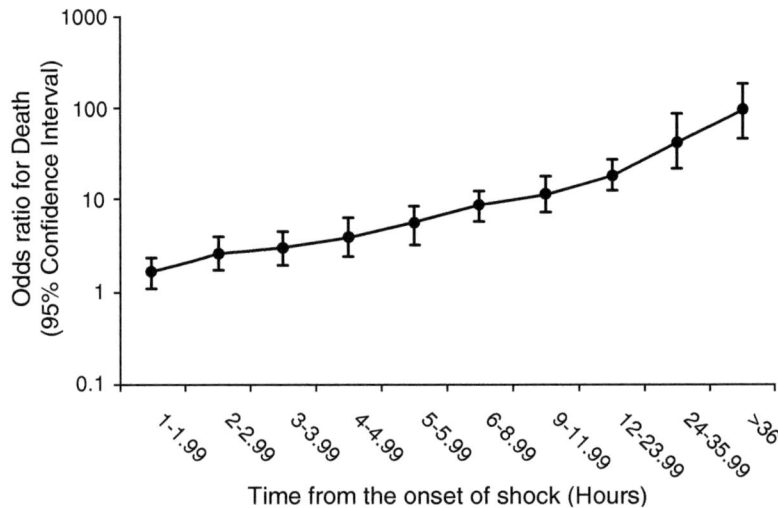

Fig. 1 The influence on in-hospital mortality of delayed initiation of antimicrobial treatment in septic shock (adapted from [13])

Table 1 Risk factors for the occurrence of multi-resistant pathogens (adapted from [35])

Previous antibiotic therapy within the last 90 days
Hospitalization for at least 5 days
High prevalence of known multi-resistant pathogens within the unit/region
Risk factors for the presence of a "healthcare-associated" pneumonia
Hospitalization for 2 days or more within the last 3 months
Residents of residential of nursing homes
Parenteral treatment at home (including antibiotics)
Chronic haemodialysis
Open-wound care at home
Family relative with evidence of colonization with multi-resistant pathogens
Immunosuppressed conditions or therapy

The major reason of ineffective initial antibiotic therapy arises from the presence of the above-highlighted resistance of the relevant pathogens. These multiresistant organisms carry an already clearly elevated mortality risk within the intensive care environment. Important risk factors for the selection of multiresistant pathogens are summarized in Table 1. Particular relevance arises in cases with preceding antibiotic exposure in the 4 weeks prior to the onset of the current infection. Narrow-spectrum antibiotics such as ampicillin and second-generation cephalosporins inherently promote resistance development much faster than broad-spectrum agents. On this basis, extended perioperative prophylaxis – before and after the day of surgery – would now, for example, be considered to be an unnecessary increase in the risk of resistance development.

With this in mind, the principles in managing severe sepsis or septic shock should be based on broad-spectrum agents, administered at high dosages (with relevant dose adaption in cases of renal or hepatic impairment). There are basically three classes of agents available (piperacillin +/− a beta-lactamase inhibitor, a pseudomonas-effective cephalosporin, or a pseudomonas-effective carbapenem). The exact dosing is shown in Table 2.

Due to the development of Gram-negative resistance of all fluoroquinolones with anti-pseudomonas properties (ciprofloxacin 3 × 400 mg or levofloxacin 2 × 500 mg), these options are no longer recommended as part of initial empirical treatment. In relation to targeted treatment, based on proven pathogenic sensitivity, these compounds remain, as before, entirely suitable. It should be noted that of all the quinolones, moxifloxacin provides the best penetration into the pulmonary compartment.

4
Monotherapy Versus Combination Therapy

Controversy remains regarding the superiority of combination therapy of antibiotics in patients with severe sepsis and septic shock. The importance of combination therapy must be assessed with consideration to the primary site of infection in the body, and the location where the infection was acquired (community or hospital acquired). While synergistic antibiotic effects have been judged as the major advantage of combination in the last few

Table 2 Initial management of severe sepsis and septic shock

Substance used as initial treatment	Daily dosages for initial treatment	Overall duration of treatment
Pseudomonas-active beta-lactams		
– Piperacillin/tazobactam	3 × 4.5 g i.v.	7–(14) days
– Cefepim or ceftazidime[a]	3 × 2.0 g i.v.	7–(14) days
– Imipenem	3 × 1.0 g i.v.	7–(14) days
– Meropenem	3 × 1.0 g i.v.	7–(14) days
Plus/minus aminoglycoside		7–10 days
Or		
Fluoroquinolone		
– Levofloxacin	2 × 500 mg i.v.	7–10 days
– Ciprofloxacin plus Pneumococcal- and S. aureus-effective antibiotic	3 × 400 mg i.v.	

[a] Given the poor efficacy of ceftazidime against –coccus infections, it is recommended in the context of empirical treatment to combine it with an effective antistaphylococcal agent

years, the current view, triggered by the emerging resistances, is that the probability to have a susceptible pathogen is higher when two antibiotics are combined, compared to only one.

For patients with sepsis caused by CAP, combination therapy with a beta-lactam antibiotic and a macrolide was shown to be superior to beta-lactam monotherapy [16]. Interestingly, combination therapy was better, even when a macrolide resistance of *S. pneumoniae* was found [17]. This suggests that perhaps anti-inflammatory properties might have had additional effects, beyond the pure antibiotic effects of macrolides. Animal models confirmed these anti-inflammatory observations [18].

For patients with VAP, there is controversy regarding combination therapy consisting of a beta-lactam and an aminoglycoside, as recommended in the various guidelines, in comparison to monotherapy. Two meta-analyses [19, 20] focusing on Gram-negative sepsis failed to identify a significant survival benefit in those patients receiving combination therapy. Indeed, detrimental effects were reported due to the high-dose aminoglycosides leading to a significant rise in the rate of renal failure. Both meta-analyses were, however, based exclusively on studies in which aminoglycosides – as previously accepted – were administered three times daily. This is nowadays considered to be inadequate dosing. Two recently published retrospective observational studies demonstrate a reduction of mortality in patients with *Pseudomonas sepsis* who were on combination therapy; however, in both studies various antibiotics and combination therapy regimens were used [21, 22].

Today once-daily administration (5–7 mg kg^{-1} body weight for gentamycin and tobramycin, 15–20 mg/kg^{-1} body weight for amikacin) is considered standard, because of the similar efficacy and fewer side effects in comparison to administration three times daily. Given the considerable side effects (oto- and nephrotoxicity), aminoglycosides should always been discontinued after 3–5 days. A recently published multicenter randomized study by the Canadian Critical Care Trials Group, comparing monotherapy treatment with meropenem with a combination therapy of meropenem and ciprofloxacin in patients with VAP, failed to demonstrate any significant benefit with combination therapy [23]. Possible limitations exist, however, in relation to the efficacy of Ciprofloxacin, given the distinct patterns of resistance in this specific situation along with its weak activity against Gram-positive organisms. In December 2007 the Sepsis Network of Excellence (SepNet) in the randomized controlled MAXSEP-Study started examining 600 patients with severe sepsis and septic shock to compare the efficacy of combination therapy (meropenem plus moxifloxacin) against meropenem monotherapy.

In patients with a sepsis focus in the abdomen, in the early phase (until day 5–7), a combination therapy with a beta-lactam antibiotic and a second antibiotic against anaerobic pathogens (metronidazol) is recommended [24]. However, it must be taken into account that many antibiotics (penicillins/inhibitor combinations, carbapenems, moxifloxacin) are active against anaerobic pathogens, therefore combination with metronidazol is not necessary.

In the late phase of intra-abdominal sepsis, enterococci, and also candida infections may play a role. Broad-spectrum penicillins and carbapenem are effective against *Enterococcus faecalis*. If these substances had been applied before, selection of *E. faecium* is possible. However, the pathogenicity of *E. faecium* is not clear. Glycopeptides or linezolid (see below) would be the treatment of choice.

At the moment, growing resistance rates of enterococci against vancomycin can be observed. Depending on the local resistances, linezolid or tigecycline should be applied. The latter is effective in the abdomen, but not approved for some pulmonary infectious. Linezolid should be combined with a beta-lactam antibiotic; tigecycline (not active against *Pseudomonas*) can only be used as monotherapy in non septic petiuts (due to low serum concentration).

For all other infections, where non-fermenters or multiresistant pathogens are suspected, the same consideration as discussed for VAP may apply.

If there is a high prevalence of MRSA, and in severe skin and soft-tissue infections, the following recommendations may be given.

5
Methicillin-Resistant *Staphylococcus aureus*

The American studies published generally employ aggressive MRSA combination therapies with glycopeptides, thereby avoiding inadequate antibiotic treatment. This can, however, only be recommended in exceptional cases, where the probability of MRSA infection related to epidemiological factors (high MRSA prevalence in the particular ward, close proximity to other MRSA-infected patients, or known MRSA colonization) in the ICU is markedly elevated. However, the principal problem is that while MRSA is (particularly in airway secretions) detected, such colonization is absolutely predictive of septic infection with these particular pathogens. On suspicion of pulmonary or skin and soft-tissue MRSA infections, sole treatment with glycopeptides (vancomycin) is not sufficient, due to poor drug concentrations in the lung. Glycopeptides must therefore be combined with an antibiotic with good tissue penetration properties (rifampicin, fosfomycin) [25]; however, the effectiveness has not been confirmed in randomized clinical studies. The effectiveness of the glycopeptides can possibly be improved by continuous infusion over 24h (1.5–2.0g vancomycin, with target serum level 16–20 mg l^{-1}), but to date only anecdotal evidence exists [26].

Alternative treatment options with oxazolidinones (linezolid) exist for severe MRSA cases – particularly those involving the pathogenic PVL-variant, causing necrotizing infections. In view of the serious neurological and hematological side effects associated with this drug, it cannot be considered as a long-term (>4 weeks) therapy. New MRSA-effective antibiotics have now been identified (tigecycline, daptomycin) with some of them already appearing in clinical studies (telavancin, ceftobiprole).

Daptomycin is a bactericidal substance and effective against Gram-positive pathogens. In staphylococcus sepsis with unknown origin, daptomycin was superior to vancomycin [27]. Daptomycin seems to be ineffective in pulmonary infections; it was inferior to ceftriaxone in a clinical trial with CAP patients [28]. In animal experiments, daptomycin appeared to be unsuitable for the treatment of pneumonia due to the inhibition of protein binding by surfactants [29]. Combination of daptomycin with broad-spectrum penicillins or with aminoglycosides has synergistic effects. Apart from pulmonary infections, daptomycin is an alternative for the treatment of sepsis.

Tigecycline is a broad-spectrum substance against Gram-positive and Gram-negative pathogens, with the exceptions of *Proteus* and *P. aeruginosa*, and is an option for the treatment of MRSA and ESBL infections. There are clinical trials with patients suffering from skin, soft-tissue, and intra-abdominal infections [30, 31]. In nosocomial pneumonia, a study presented at the American Conference for Infectious Diseases revealed no improved efficacy against MRSA infection compared with vancomycin. Perhaps tigecycline must be given in much higher doses than currently believed. Tigecycline is bacteriostatic, and in severe sepsis and septic shock, the substance should be combined with another bactericidal antibiotic. However, to date, there are no data from combination studies.

6
Treatment Failure

The lack of clinical improvement within 48–72 h of beginning treatment should be considered as treatment failure. A change in therapy to an antibiotic from a different class (i.e., from cephalosporin to carbapanem, or from the latter to a fluoroquinolone) is indicated at this stage. Alternatively, for cases initially treated with monotherapy, the subsequent initiation of combination treatment should be considered.

If there is no improvement in the clinical condition despite these changes, alternative causative organisms must be considered (fungal infections, so-called atypical bacteria such as *Legionella* or *Chlamydia*) or the involvement of resistant-pathogens such as MRSA or ESBL. It should also be remembered that antibiotics can only work at the sites where they are delivered to. Persistent pyrexia can result from cavity infections (such as lung empyemas, intra-abdominal abscesses and endocarditis), which can be clinically difficult to recognize.

In cases of prolonged antibiotic treatment with discrepancies between the clinical symptoms and inflammatory indices, consideration should be given to the possibility of an antibiotic-associated so-called "drug fever" as the underlying cause. In this specific situation, and if the clinical condition allows, a temporary cessation of treatment for 24–48 h may be worthwhile. If the antibiotic is responsible, an improvement in the fever will generally follow within 24–36 h of treatment cessation.

Relationships between the excessive use of antibiotics and the subsequent development of resistance in important pathogens against these substances are clear [32]. Attempts have therefore been made to reduce the resistance rate by regularly changing the primary antibiotic administered. The first studies on this strategy demonstrated not only a decline in the resistance rate, but also, somewhat surprisingly, a lower general rate of infections as well as improved survival [33]. However, subsequent and more elaborately designed studies could not confirm these findings [34].

7
Implications for Clinical Practice

It is now well documented that delayed diagnosis, along with delayed or incorrect antibiotic treatment, reduces the probability of patient survival. On the other hand over-use of these drugs has resulted in the development of resistance against the most important antibiotics. The initiation of a broad-spectrum, high-dose empirical therapy in patients exhibiting severe sepsis and septic shock must occur immediately after the diagnosis is established and should not be delayed pending microbiological results. Initial treatment choices should always take into account local patterns of resistance, and treatment should be subsequently adjusted on receipt of relevant microbiological findings. The duration of treatment is determined by the type of infection, the pathogens detected, as well as the clinical response of the patient to treatment. Treatment should continue until clinical success is apparent and terminated as soon as possible thereafter.

Combination therapy is established for severe infections and based on the results of clinical trials (endocarditis, toxic shock syndrome, CAP). The major goal for combination therapy is to conquer resistances. Depending on the microbiologic results and the clinical success, de-escalation to monotherapy should be tried after 3–5 days.

With the background of increasing resistances against antibiotics, clinical trials for combination therapy, e.g., for MRSA infections or fungal sepsis, are necessary, to base the current practice on better knowledge.

References

1. Alberti C, Brun-Buisson C, Chevret S, Antonelli M, Goodman SV, Martin C, Moreno R, Ochagavia AR, Palazzo M, Werdan K, Le Gall JR. European Sepsis Study Group. Systemic inflammatory response and progression to severe sepsis in critically ill infected patients. Am J Respir Crit Care Med 2005; 171(5):461–468
2. Angus DC, Linde-Zwirble WT, Lidicker J, Clermont G, Carcillo J, Pinsky MR. Epidemiology of severe sepsis in the United States: analysis of incidence, outcome and associated cost of care. Crit Care Med 2001; 29:1303–1310
3. Brun-Boisson C, Roudot-Thoraval F, Girou E, Grennier-Sennelier E, Durand-Saleski I. The cost of sepsissyndromes in the intensive care unit and influence of hospital acquired sepsis. Intens Care Med 2003; 29:1464–1471
4. Engel C, Brunkhorst FM, Bone HG, Brunkhorst R, Gerlach H, Grond S, Gruendling M, Huhle G, Jaschinski U, John S, Mayer K, Oppert M, Olthoff D, Quintel M, Ragaller M, Rossaint R,

Stuber F, Weiler N, Welte T, Bogatsch H, Hartog C, Loeffler M, Reinhart K. Epidemiology of sepsis in Germany: results from a national prospective multicenter study. Intens Care Med 2007; 33(4):606–618. Epub 2007 Feb 24
5. Osmon S, Warren D, Seiler SM, Shannon W, Fraser VJ, Kollef MH. The influence of infection on hospital mortality for patients requiring > 48h of intensive care. Chest 2003; 124(3):1021–1029
6. Martin GS, Mannino DM, Eaton S, Moss M. The epidemiology of sepsis in the United States from 1979 through 2000. N Engl J Med 2003; 348:1546–1554
7. Martin GS, Mannino DM, Eaton S, Moss M. The epidemiology of sepsis in the United States from 1979 through 2000. N Engl J Med 2003; 17; 348(16):1546–1554
8. Namias N, Samiian L, Nino D, Shirazi E, O'Neill K, Kett DH, Ginzburg E, McKenney MG, Sleeman D, Cohn SM. Incidence and susceptibility of pathogenic bacteria vary between intensive care units within a single hospital: implications for empiric antibiotic strategies. J Trauma 2000; 49(4):638–645
9. Meyer E, Schwab F, Jonas D, Rhüden H, Gastmeier P, Daschner FD. Temporal changes in bacterial resistance in German intensive care units, 2001–2003: data from the SARI (surveillance of antimicrobial use and antimicrobial resistance in intensive care units) project. J Hosp Infect 2005; 60(4):348–352
10. Loo VG, Poirier L, Miller MA, Oughton M, Libman MD, Michaud S, Bourgault AM, Nguyen T, Frenette C, Kelly M, Vibien A, Brassard P, Fenn S, Dewar K, Hudson TJ, Horn R, Rene P, Monczak Y, Dascal A. A predominantly clonal multi-institutional outbreak of *Clostridium difficile*-associated diarrhea with high morbidity and mortality. N Engl J Med 2005; 353(23):2442–2449
11. Bartlett JG. Clinical practice. Antibiotic-associated diarrhea. N Engl J Med 2002; 346(5):334–339
12. Valles J, Rello J, Ochagavia A, Garnacho J, Alcala MA. Community-acquired bloodstream infection in critically ill adult patients: impact of shock and inappropriate antibiotic therapy on survival. Chest 2003; 123(5):1615–1624
13. Kumar A, Roberts D, Wood KE, Light B, Parrillo JE, Sharma S, Suppes R, Feinstein D, Zanotti S, Taiberg L, Gurka D, Kumar A, Cheang M. Duration of hypotension before initiation of effective antimicrobial therapy is the critical determinant of survival in human septic shock. Crit Care Med 2006; 34(6):1589–1596
14. Blot SI, Rodriguez A, Solé-Violán J, Blanquer J, Almirall J, Rello J. Effects of delayed oxygenation assessment on time to antibiotic delivery and mortality in patients with severe community-acquired pneumonia. Community-Acquired Pneumonia Intensive Care Units (CAPUCI) Study Investigators. Crit Care Med 2007; 35(11):2509–2514
15. Alberti C, Brun-Buisson C, Burchardi H et al. Epidemiology of sepsis and infection in ICU patients from an international multicentre cohort study. Intens Care Med 2002; 28:108–121
16. Rodríguez A, Mendia A, Sirvent JM, Barcenilla F, de la Torre-Prados MV, Solé-Violán J, Rello J. CAPUCI Study Group. Combination antibiotic therapy improves survival in patients with community-acquired pneumonia and shock. Crit Care Med 2007; 35(6):1493–1498
17. Restrepo MI, Mortensen EM, Waterer GW, Wunderink RG, Coalson JJ, Anzueto A. Impact of macrolide therapy on mortality for patients with severe sepsis due to pneumonia. Eur Respir J 2009; 33(1):153–159
18. Karlström A, Boyd KL, English BK, McCullers JA. Treatment with protein synthesis inhibitors improves outcomes of secondary bacterial pneumonia after influenza. J Infect Dis 2009; 199(3):311–319
19. Paul M, Benuri-Silbiger I, Soares-Weiser K, Leibovici L. Beta lactam monotherapy versus beta lactam-aminoglycoside combination therapy for sepsis in immunocompetent patients: systematic review and meta-analysis of randomised trials. BMJ 2004; 328(7441):668
20. Safdar N, Handelsman J, Maki DG. Does combination antimicrobial therapy reduce mortality in Gram-negative bacteraemia? A meta-analysis. Lancet Infect Dis 2004; 4(8):519–527

21. Chamot E, Boffi El Amari E, Rohner P, Van Delden C. Effectiveness of combination antimicrobial therapy for *Pseudomonas aeruginosa* bacteremia. Antimicrob Agents Chemother 2003; 47(9):2756–2764
22. Garnacho-Montero J, Sa-Borges M, Sole-Violan J, Barcenilla F, Escoresca-Ortega A, Ochoa M, Cayuela A, Rello J. Optimal management therapy for *Pseudomonas aeruginosa* ventilator-associated pneumonia: an observational, multicenter study comparing monotherapy with combination antibiotic therapy. Crit Care Med 2007; 35(8):1888–1895
23. Canadian Critical Care Trials Group; Heyland D, Dodek P, Muscedere J, Day A. A randomized trial of diagnostic techniques for ventilator-associated pneumonia. New Engl J Med 2006; 355(25):2619–2630
24. Dellinger RP, Levy MM, Carlet JM, Bion J, Parker MM, Jaeschke R, Reinhart K, Angus DC, Brun-Buisson C, Beale R, Calandra T, Dhainaut JF, Gerlach H, Harvey M, Marini JJ, Marshall J, Ranieri M, Ramsay G, Sevransky J, Thompson BT, Townsend S, Vender JS, Zimmerman JL, Vincent JL. Surviving Sepsis Campaign: international guidelines for management of severe sepsis and septic shock: 2008. Intens Care Med 2008; 34(1):17–60
25. Burkhardt O, Derendorf H, Welte T. Neue Antibiotika für die Behandlung von MRSA-Infektionen. Med Monatsschr Pharm 2006; 29(2):56–62
26. Rello J, Sole-Violan J, Sa-Borges M, Garnacho-Montero J, Munoz E, Sirgo G, Olona M, Diaz E. Pneumonia caused by oxacillin-resistant *Staphylococcus aureus* treated with glycopeptides. Crit Care Med 2005; 33(9):1983–1987
27. Fowler VG Jr, Boucher HW, Corey GR, Abrutyn E, Karchmer AW, Rupp ME, Levine DP, Chambers HF, Tally FP, Vigliani GA, Cabell CH, Link AS, DeMeyer I, Filler SG, Zervos M, Cook P, Parsonnet J, Bernstein JM, Price CS, Forrest GN, Fätkenheuer G, Gareca M, Rehm SJ, Brodt HR, Tice A, Cosgrove SE; S. aureus Endocarditis and Bacteremia Study Group. Daptomycin versus standard therapy for bacteremia and endocarditis caused by Staphylococcus aureus. N Engl J Med 2006; 355(7):653–665
28. Pertel PE, Bernardo P, Fogarty C, Matthews P, Northland R, Benvenuto M, Thorne GM, Luperchio SA, Arbeit RD, Alder J. Effects of prior effective therapy on the efficacy of daptomycin and ceftriaxone for the treatment of community-acquired pneumonia. Clin Infect Dis 2008; 46(8):1142–1151
29. Silverman JA, Mortin LI, Vanpraagh AD, Li T, Alder J. Inhibition of daptomycin by pulmonary surfactant: in vitro modeling and clinical impact. J Infect Dis 2005; 191(12):2149–2152
30. Ellis-Grosse EJ, Babinchak T, Dartois N, Rose G, Loh E; Tigecycline 300 cSSSI Study Group; Tigecycline 305 cSSSI Study Group. The efficacy and safety of tigecycline in the treatment of skin and skin-structure infections: results of 2 double-blind phase 3 comparison studies with vancomycin-aztreonam. Clin Infect Dis 2005; 41(Suppl 5):S341–S353
31. Babinchak T, Ellis-Grosse E, Dartois N, Rose GM, Loh E; Tigecycline 301 Study Group; Tigecycline 306 Study Group. The efficacy and safety of tigecycline for the treatment of complicated intra-abdominal infections: analysis of pooled clinical trial data. Clin Infect Dis 2005; 41(Suppl 5):S354–S3567
32. Neuhauser MM, Weinstein RA, Rydman R, Danziger LH, Karam G, Quinn JP. Antibiotic resistance among gram-negative bacilli in US intensive care units: implications for fluoroquinolone use. JAMA 2003; 289(7):885–888
33. Gruson D, Hilbert G, Vargas F, Valentino R, Bui N, Pereyre S, Bebear C, Bebear CM, Gbikpi-Benissan G. Strategy of antibiotic rotation: long-term effect on incidence and susceptibilities of Gram-negative bacilli responsible for ventilator-associated pneumonia. Crit Care Med 2003; 31(7):1908–1914
34. van Loon HJ, Vriens MR, Fluit AC, Troelstra A, van der Werken C, Verhoef J, Bonten MJ. Antibiotic rotation and development of gram-negative antibiotic resistance. Am J Respir Crit Care Med 2005; 171(5):480–487

35. American Thoracic Society; Infectious Diseases Society of America. Guidelines for the management of adults with hospital-acquired, ventilator-associated, and healthcare-associated pneumonia. Am J Respir Crit Care Med 2005; 171(4):388–416
36. Dellinger RP, Carlet JM, Masur H, Gerlach H, Calandra T, Cohen J, Gea-Banachloche J, Keh D, Marshall JC, Parker MM, Ramsey Gzimmermann JL, Vincent JL, Levy MM. Surviving sepsis campaign guidelines for management of severe sepsis and septic shock. Intens Care Med 2004; 30:536–555

Index

A
Activated protein C (APC), 32, 133, 137–140
Acute Dialysis Quality Initiative (ADQI), 99
Acute kidney injury (AKI). *See also* Acute renal failure (ARF)
  definition and stratification
    AKIN classification, 100
    glomerular filtration rate (GFR), 99
    RIFLE classification, 99–100
  diagnosis and monitoring
    conventional biomarkers, 100
    GFR and Cr_s relationship, 101
  management, 106
  monitoring and diagnostic tests
    blood urea nitrogen (BUN), 102
    diagnostic algorithm, 103
    renal biopsy, 103
    sodium fractional excretion, 103
    ultrasonography (US), 102
  new biomarkers, 101–102
  prevention
    contrast-induced nephropathy risk score, 105
    contrast related nephrotoxicity (CRN), 106
    intraabdominal hypertension (IAH), 104
    ischemic renal failure, 103
    other preventive actions, 106
    prerenal disease and renal ischemic damage, differences, 103
    pulmonary artery catheter (PAC), 104
    toxic renal failure, 104–106
  sepsis, 98
Acute kidney injury network (AKIN), 100
Acute Physiology and Chronic Health Evaluation (APACHE) II score, 59, 60
Acute renal failure (ARF), 55, 59, 97–101, 106, 110
Acute renal injury, extracorporeal blood purification
  AKI and sepsis, 98
  AKI prevention, 103–106
  definition and stratification, 98–100
  diagnosis and monitoring, 100–103
  management, 106–112
Acute respiratory distress syndrome (ARDS), 7, 33, 34, 56, 59
Acute tubular necrosis (ATN), 97, 103
Adjunctive therapy, 61
ADQI. *See* Acute Dialysis Quality Initiative
AKIN. *See* Acute kidney injury network
American College of Chest Physicians (ACCP), 11
American Thoracic Society (ATS), 54, 59
Antibiotics
  clindamycin, 27
  combination, 27–28
  macrolides, 27, 28
  penicillin, 26, 27
  severe sepsis
    clinical practice implications, 155
    epidemiology and microbiology, 147–148
    methicillin-resistant *Staphylococcus aureus*, 153–154
    monotherapy *vs.* combination therapy, 151–153
    resistance development, 148–149
    treatment, 149–151, 154–155
Antimicrobial therapy
  delay, 66–67
  fluorescence in situ hybridization (FISH), 68
  hybridization approach, 67, 70, 78
  limitations, 77
Antithrombin (AT), 133, 136–137

APACHE. *See* Acute Physiology and Chronic Health Evaluation
APC. *See* Activated protein C
Appropriate antibiotic treatment, 59
Appropriateness of initial empirical antibiotic therapy, 43
ARDS. *See* Acute respiratory distress syndrome
ATN. *See* Acute tubular necrosis
ATS. *See* American Thoracic Society

B
Bacteremia, 27–28, 30, 52, 55–57
Biomarkers, 43, 55, 59
  C-reactive protein, 43
  procalcitonin, 43
Blood culture, 66–72, 74–78
Bloodstream infections (BSIs), 66

C
Cancer, 2–3, 7–8
Candida, 7
CAP PIRO score, 55–61
Chronic obstructive pulmonary disease (COPD), 52, 53, 55, 57
  corticosteroids, 25
Community-acquired pneumonia (CAP)
  bacteremic pneumococcal pneumonia, 58
  pneumococcal bacteremic pneumonia, 53
  severe CAP, 51, 52, 55–60
Comorbidities, 52, 55–57
Confusion, urea, respiratory rate, blood pressure, age ≥ 65 years (CURB-65), 53, 54
Continuous hemodiafiltration, 34
Continuous renal replacement therapy (CRRT), 107, 108, 110, 111
Contrast-related nephrotoxicity (CRN), 106
COPD. *See* Chronic obstructive pulmonary disease
Cortisol, 59
C-reactive protein (CRP), 1, 59
CRP. *See* C-reactive protein
CRRT. *See* Continuous renal replacement therapy
CURB-65. *See* Confusion, urea, respiratory rate, blood pressure, age ≥ 65 years
Cytokines, 59

D
28-Day mortality, 59
Disseminated intravascular coagulation (DIC), 131–132, 134, 136, 138, 140

E
Early goal-directed therapy, 32–33
Endothelial protein C receptor (EPCR), 133, 137–138, 140
Escherichia (E.) coli, 134
Extracorporeal purification treatments (EPT), 107, 108, 110, 111

F
Fibrinolysis, 113, 138

G
Genetic, 24–25
  CD14, 25
  TLR, 25
  tumor necrosis factor (TNF), 25
Glomerular filtration rate (GFR), 99, 100, 102, 104
Granulocyte colony-stimulating factor (G-CSF), 29, 30

H
Heparin, 136–137
Host response, 40, 43, 55, 58, 59
  acute renal failure, 43
  shock, 43
  systolic blood pressure, 43
Hypoxemia, 29, 55, 58

I
ICU. *See* Intensive Care Unit; Intensive care units
IDSA. *See* Infectious diseases Society of America
Immune Response, 3–6
Immunity, 117–118, 120, 122–123
Immunization, 57
Immunocompromise, 55–57, 60
Immunoglobulin(s), 118, 120, 123–126
Immunosuppression, 52
Infection, 1–5, 7
Infectious Diseases Society of America (IDSA), 54

Inflammation, 55, 58
Insult, 55, 57–58
Insult/infection, 40, 42–43
  Acinetobacter baumannii, 42
  bacteremia, 42
  early-onset VAP, 42
  high-risk microorganisms, 42
  late-onset VAP, 42
  microorganism virulence, 42
  MRSA, 43
  Pseudomonas aeruginosa, 42
Intensive care units (ICUs), 11, 39–44
Intensive respiratory and hemodynamic support, 58
Intravenous immunoglobulins (IVIC), 28

L
Lipopolysaccharide (LPS), 134–140
Logistic organ dysfunction (LOD) system, 13
Lower respiratory tract infection, 40

M
Macrolides, 58
Mechanical ventilation, 52, 54, 57, 60
Methicillin-resistant *Staphylococcus aureus* (MRSA), 71
Microparticles (MPs), 132, 134–135
MODS. *See* Multiple organ dysfunction/ failure syndrome
Mortality, 40–47, 51–53, 57–60
Multiple organ dysfunction, 51
Multiple organ dysfunction/failure scores
  logical boxes, 14
  multivariate analysis, 15
  simplified acute physiology score (SAPS), 14
  systemic inflammatory response syndrome (SIRS), 14
Multiple organ dysfunction/failure syndrome (MODS), 12

N
Noninvasive Mechanical Ventilation (NIMV), 33
Nosocomial infection, 39, 40

O
Older patients, 57
One PIRO or many PIROs, 15–18

computation scoresheet, 16–18
ventilator-associated pneumonia (VAP-PIRO), 15
Organ dysfunction, 1–4, 6–7, 39, 40, 44, 51, 55, 59
  ARDS, 43
Organ dysfunction/failure scores, 12–14
  logistic organ dysfunction (LOD) system, 12
  pressure-adjusted heart rate or PAR, 13
Organ failure, 59–60

P
PAC. *See* Pulmonary artery catheter
PAI-1. *See* Plasminogen activator inhibitor type-1
Panton-Valentine leukocidin, 58
PAR. *See* Pressure-adjusted heart rate; Protease-activated receptor
Pathogenesis, 58
PCR. *See* Polymerase chain reaction
PC. *See* Protein C
PIRO, 23–34, 39–47
  concept, 55, 57
PIRO/MODS scores
  nosocomial *vs.* community-acquired infection, 18–19
  surviving sepsis campaign, 18
Plasminogen activator inhibitor type-1 (PAI-1), 133, 138–139
Platelets, 135
Pneumococcal conjugated vaccine
  effectiveness, 89, 90
  herd immunity effect, 89, 94
  replacement phenomenon, 90, 95
Pneumococcal polysaccharide vaccine
  immunological response, 88, 90
  revaccination, 89
Pneumonia, 119–123, 125
Pneumonia severity index (PSI), 53, 54, 60
Polymerase chain reaction (PCR), broad range, 70
Predisposition, 3–4, 7, 40–42, 44, 55–57
  age, 41, 42
  chronic heart failure, 41
  chronic hepatopathy, 41, 42
  Chronic obstructive pulmonary disease (COPD), 41
  immune system deficiency, 41
  trauma, 41
Pressure-adjusted heart rate (PAR), 13

Prevention, 23, 24
  immunization, 24
  nutrition, 24
  smoking, 25
  vaccination, 23, 25, 26
Procalcitonin, 1, 5, 59
Protease-activated receptors (PARs), 132, 139–140
Protein C (PC), 132, 137–138
PSI. *See* Pneumonia severity index
Pulmonary artery catheter (PAC), 104

Q
Quantitative real-time polymerase chain reaction, 58

R
Radiological infiltrates, 58
Real time PCR
  available systems, 75–76
  contamination, 74–75
  interpretation, 77–78
  limitations, 78
  pathogen discrimination, 70
Renal replacement therapies
  acute renal failure
    continuous renal replacement therapy (CRRT), 107
    continuous venovenous hemodiafiltration (CVVHF), 109
    dialytrauma, 110
    dynamic approach to extracorporeal purification treatments, 109
    slow low-efficient daily dialysis (SLEDD), 108
  sepsis and MODS
    controversial aspects, HVHF, 112
    mean arterial pressure (MAP), 110
    putative mechanisms, 111–112
Resolution, 43
Response, 55, 58–59

S
SAPS. *See* Simplified acute physiology score
SCCM. *See* Society of Critical Care Medicine
Score, 39–47
  Acute Physiology and Chronic Health Evaluation (APACHE II), 39–44
  multiple organ dysfunction score (MODS), 39
  organ dysfunction and infection score (ODIN), 39
  sequential organ failure assessment (SOFA), 39
  simplified acute physiology score (SAPS), 39
Sepsis, 117, 119–120, 125–126
  severe sepsis, 51, 52, 55, 58
Sepsis-related organ failure assessment (SOFA), 13, 14
Septic shock, 51, 52, 54, 55, 57, 58
Sequential organ failure assessment (SOFA), 6
Severe CAP, 51, 52, 55–60
Severe sepsis, risk stratification
  multiple organ dysfunction/failure scores, 14–15
  one PIRO or many PIROs, 15–18
  organ dysfunction/failure scores, 12–14
  PIRO/MODS scores, 18–19
Sex, 3, 4
Shock, refractory, 59
Simplified acute physiology score (SAPS), 14, 15, 18, 19
SIRS. *See* Systemic inflammatory response syndrome
SMART-COP, 54, 55
Society of Critical Care Medicine (SCCM), 11
SOFA score, 59
SOFA. *See* Sequential organ failure assessment; Sepsis-related organ failure assessment
Staphylococcus aureus, MRSA, 58
Steroids, 59
Streptococcus pneumoniae, 68, 71, 73
  clinical differences, 91–94
  DNA, 58
  high invasive disease potential, 92–93
  immunization, 88–91
  low invasive disease potential, 93–94
  mortality, 87, 91–94
  pediatric serotypes, 91
  polysaccharide capsule, 87
  serotypes, 87–95
Systemic inflammatory response syndrome (SIRS), 1, 14, 65, 76
Systemic vascular resistance (SVR), 1

T
Thrombin, 132–137, 139–140
Thrombomodulin (TM), 133, 137

Tissue factor pathway inhibitor (TFPI), 133, 136
Tissue factor (TF), 132–134, 136
Tumor, lymph nodes, metastasis (TNM), 23
Tumor necrosis factor (TNF), 4
Tumor necrosis factor-α (TNF-α), 133, 134

V

Ventilator-associated pneumonia (VAP), 7, 15, 39
Ventilator-associated pneumonia PIRO score (VAP PIRO), 39–47
   comorbidities, 44
von Willebrand factor (vWF), 133, 135

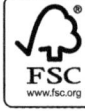

MIX
Papier aus verantwortungsvollen Quellen
Paper from responsible sources
FSC® C105338

If you have any concerns about our products,
you can contact us on
ProductSafety@springernature.com

In case Publisher is established outside the EU,
the EU authorized representative is:
**Springer Nature Customer Service Center GmbH
Europaplatz 3, 69115 Heidelberg, Germany**

Printed by Libri Plureos GmbH
in Hamburg, Germany